ABC OF
INTENSIVE CARE

ABC OF
INTENSIVE CARE

Edited by

MERVYN SINGER

Reader in Intensive Care Medicine, Bloomsbury Institute of Intensive Care Medicine,
University College London, London

and

IAN GRANT

Director of Intensive Care, Western General Hospital, Edinburgh

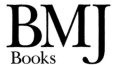

First published in 1999
Second impression 2002
Third impression 2004
by BMJ Books, BMA House, Tavistock Square,
London WC1H 9JR

www.bmjbooks.com

British Library Cataloguing in Publication Data

A catalogue record for this book is available from the
British Library

ISBN 0-7279-1436-7

Typeset by Apek Typesetters, Nailsea, Bristol
Printed and bound by Craft Print Ltd, Singapore

Contents

Contributors

Sheila Adam
Clinical Nurse Specialist, Intensive Care Unit, University College London Hospitals, London

Peter JD Andrews
Consultant, Western General Hospital, Edinburgh

David Bennett
Professor of Intensive Care Medicine, St George's Hospital Medical School, London

Julian Bion
Reader in Intensive Care Medicine, Queen Elizabeth Medical Centre, Birmingham

Simon Cohen
Senior Lecturer in Intensive Care, University College London Hospitals, London

Alan Cumming
Consultant Nephrologist, Edinburgh Royal Infirmary, Edinburgh

Timothy W Evans
Professor of Intensive Care Medicine, Imperial College School of Medicine, Royal Brompton Hospital, London

Sally Forrest
Superintendent Physiotherapist, University College London Hospitals, London

Ian S Grant
Director of Intensive Care, Western General Hospital, Edinburgh

Richard D Griffiths
Reader in Medicine, Intensive Care Research Group (Whiston Hospital), Department of Medicine, University of Liverpool, Liverpool

Kevin Gunning
Consultant in Anaesthesia and Intensive Care, John Farman Intensive Care Unit, Addenbrooke's Hospital, Cambridge

C J Hinds
Senior Lecturer in Anaesthesia and Intensive Care Medicine, St Bartholomew's and the Royal London School of Medicine, Queen Mary and Westfield College, London

Christina Jones
Research Associate, Intensive Care Research Group (Whiston Hospital), Department of Medicine, University of Liverpool, Liverpool

Rod Little
Professor, North West Injury Research Centre, University of Manchester, Manchester

Mick Nielsen
Director of the General Intensive Care Unit, Southampton General Hospital, Southampton

Peter Nightingale
Director of Intensive Care, Withington Hospital, Manchester

Saxon A Ridley
Director of Intensive Care, Norfolk and Norwich Hospital, Norwich

Kathy Rowan
Scientific Director, Intensive Care National Audit Research Centre, London

Maire P Shelly
Consultant in Anaesthesia and Intensive Care, Withington Hospital, Manchester

Alasdair Short
Director of Intensive Care, Broomfield Hospital, Chelmsford, Essex

Mervyn Singer
Reader in Intensive Care Medicine, Bloomsbury Institute of Intensive Care Medicine, University College London, London

Cary Smith
Director of Intensive Care Medicine, Queen Alexandra Hospital, Portsmouth

Mark Smithies
Director of Intensive Care, University Hospital of Wales, Cardiff

Peter GM Wallace
Consultant Anaesthetist, Western Infirmary, Glasgow

D Watson
Senior Lecturer in Anaesthesia and Intensive Care Medicine, St Bartholomew's and the Royal London School of Medicine, Queen Mary and Westfield College, London

Bob Winter
Consultant in Intensive Care, University Hospital, Nottingham

Introduction

Intensive care as a specialty has developed from nothing in less than 50 years. Its origins stem from the successful use of positive pressure ventilation to treat respiratory failure due to poliomyelitis in Copenhagen in 1952. Similar improvements occurred in the outcome of patients with severe closed chest injuries; mortality decreased from 76% to 16% in patients treated in Edinburgh between 1955 and 1965 as a result both of positive pressure ventilation, and the opening of an assisted ventilation unit, an innovation mirrored across the world in the 1950s and 60s.

Treatment of respiratory failure, coupled by simultaneous advances in cardiovascular resuscitation led not only to patient survival in many cases, but also to the syndrome of multiple organ dysfunction or failure, where a patient had simultaneous dysfunction of more than one organ, with death frequently only being delayed.

The assisted ventilation unit metamorphosed into the intensive care unit where expertise and equipment were gathered for the monitoring and support of organ system function, including the pulmonary artery catheter for cardiovascular monitoring, haemodialysis and then haemofiltration for renal replacement therapy, and parenteral nutrition for those with gastro-intestinal failure.

As these developments took place, the Intensive Care Society was established in the United Kingdom in 1970 to bring together clinicians whose main interest was caring for critically ill patients. Similar societies have since been established in most other countries, including the Society of Critical Care Medicine in the USA, and across continents (e.g. the European Society of Intensive Care Medicine). It is noteworthy that the ICS from its beginning had a multi-specialty membership, and it should be stressed that intensive care remains a multidisciplinary specialty which requires close cooperation of specialists from many fields.

Over the past 25 years progress in understanding the pathophysiological basis of critical illness, technological developments and therapeutic advances have been rapid. The effects of more aggressive medical and surgical treatment in an ever older and sicker population have led to increased numbers of candidates for intensive care, but the increasing costs of care have meant that resources have not increased to meet demand. Furthermore, the existence of 'mechanical life support' has exposed ethical issues such as prolongation of life and, conversely, withdrawal of treatment.

The ICU is now a pivotal component of the modern acute hospital. Expertise developed in ICU underpins many of the emergency medical services of the hospital, including resuscitation teams and high dependency care. It has become very clear in recent years that specialist training of the intensive care doctor is essential; in the UK this has recently led to the recognition of intensive care medicine as a specialty in its own right, with the introduction of intensive care specialists with joint accreditation in intensive care medicine and their parent specialty (anaesthesia, medicine, surgery). The intensive care specialist has expertise in acute aspects of most specialties, practising holistic medicine, and treating organ dysfunction in the context of overall function.

Publication of the *ABC of Intensive Care* comes, therefore, at a very opportune time when our specialty is coming of age. We hope that we have provided background knowledge to doctors and other healthcare professionals who have patients requiring intensive care, but who do not necessarily work directly in an ICU.

We have explained the organisation of an ICU and discussed who would benefit from intensive care. Intensive care support of the various failing organ systems is also covered. We have stressed the role of a variety of professions involving nurses and physiotherapists in the holistic care of the critically ill patient. Ethical issues are aired and the recovery phase is described to help readers understand the ordeal the long-term ICU patient has gone through and, perhaps continues to suffer from. We have balanced more scientific areas such as organ dysfunction, and severity scoring with practical guidelines for transport of the critically ill, an area of medicine which extends out with the speciality of intensive care. It is recognised that doctors pursuing careers in acute specialties such as anaesthesia, medicine and surgery should be familiar with the principles of managing critically ill patients, and should rotate to intensive care for that training. The publication of the *ABC of Intensive Care* is intended to make the reader, either those undergoing training in or whose specialities interface with intensive care, aware of the scope and philosophy of ICU management.

Mervyn Singer
Ian Grant

1 Organisation of intensive care

David Bennett, Julian Bion

Intensive care dates from the polio epidemic in Copenhagen in 1952. Doctors reduced the 90% mortality in patients receiving respiratory support with the cuirass ventilator to 40% by a combination of manual positive pressure ventilation provided through a tracheostomy by medical students and by caring for patients in a specific area of the hospital instead of across different wards. Having an attendant continuously at the bedside improved the quality of care but increased the costs and, in some cases, death was merely delayed.

These findings are still relevant to intensive care today, even though it has expanded enormously so that almost every hospital will have some form of intensive care unit. Many questions still remain unanswered regarding the relation between costs and quality of intensive care, the size and location of intensive care units, the number of nursing and medical staff and intensive care beds required, and how to direct scarce resources towards those most likely to benefit.

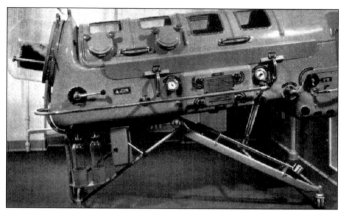

The origins of intensive care can be traced to the 1952 polio epidemic in Copenhagen

Patients

Intensive care beds are occupied by patients with a wide range of clinical conditions but all have dysfunction or failure of one or more organs, particularly respiratory and cardiovascular systems. Patients usually require intensive monitoring, and most need some form of mechanical or pharmacological support such as mechanical ventilation, renal replacement therapy, or vasoactive drugs. As patients are admitted from every department in the hospital, staff in intensive care need to have a broad range of clinical experience and a holistic approach to patient care.

The length of patient stay varies widely. Most patients are discharged within 1-2 days, commonly after postoperative respiratory and cardiovascular support and monitoring. Some patients, however, may require support for several weeks or months. These patients often have multiple organ dysfunction. Overall mortality in intensive care is 20-30%, with a further 10% dying on the ward after discharge from intensive care.

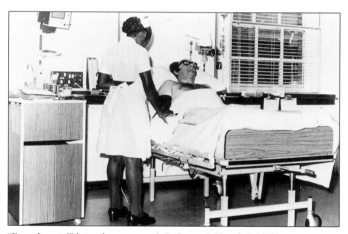

"Experimental" intensive care ward, St George's Hospital, 1967

Provision

Intensive care comprises 1-2% of total bed numbers in the United Kingdom; this compares with proportions as high as 20% in the United States. Patients admitted in Britain therefore tend be more severely ill than those in America. The average intensive care unit in Britain has four to six beds, although units in larger hospitals, especially those receiving tertiary referrals, are bigger. Few units have more than 15 beds. Throughput varies from below 200 to over 1500 patients a year. In addition to general intensive care units, specialty beds are provided for cardiothoracic, neurosurgical, paediatric, and neonatal patients in regional centres.

The frequent shortages of intensive care beds and recent expansion of high dependency units have led to renewed efforts to define criteria for admission and discharge and standards of service provision. Strict categorisation is difficult; an agitated, confused but otherwise stable patient often requires at least as much attention as a sedated, mechanically ventilated patient. Furthermore, underresourced hospitals may have to refuse admission to those who would otherwise be admitted. A recent study sponsored by the Department of Health suggested that

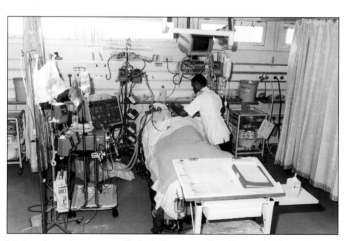

Modern intensive care usually includes comprehensive monitoring and organ support. Pressure on resources is high

patients refused intensive care have a higher mortality than similar patients who do get admitted.

Transfer to another hospital is generally reserved for those patients requiring mechanical ventilation, renal support, or specialist treatment not available in the referring hospital. Transfer of such critically ill patients is not undertaken lightly. It is labour intensive and should be performed by experienced staff with specialised equipment. In addition, such transfers remove staff from the referring hospital, often at times when they are in short supply.

Staffing

Medical
Each intensive care unit has several consultants (ranging from two to seven) with responsibility for clinical care, one of whom will be the clinical director. There are few full time intensivists in the United Kingdom. Most consultants will have anaesthetic or medical sessions in addition to their intensive care commitments. The consultants provide 24 hour non-resident cover.

In general, junior doctor staffing levels are lower in Britain than elsewhere in Europe. Most junior doctors are either anaesthetic senior house officers or specialist registrars, who may provide dedicated cover to the intensive care unit or have duties in other clinical areas such as obstetrics and emergency theatre. Increasingly, posts are being incorporated into medical or surgical rotations. Larger units often also have a more senior registrar on a longer attachment. These are training posts for those intending to become fully accredited intensivists. Such training schemes are a relatively recent innovation in Britain.

The medical staff will typically perform a morning ward round and a less formal round in the afternoon. The on call team does a further round in the evening.

Nursing
The general policy in the United Kingdom is to allocate one nurse to each intensive care patient at all times with two or three shifts a day. One nurse may care for two less sick patients, and occasionally a particularly sick patient may require two nurses. This nurse:patient ratio requires up to seven established nursing posts for each bed and an average of 30-50 nurses per unit. Elsewhere in Europe the nurse:patient ratio is usually 1:2 or 1:3, although the units are larger and have a higher proportion of low risk patients. Many intensive care nurses will have completed a specialist training programme and have extensive experience and expertise. Not surprisingly, nursing salaries comprise the largest component of the intensive care budget. However, a shortage exists of appropriately qualified staff, which leads to refused admissions, cancellation of major elective operations, and a heavy and stressful workload for the existing nurses. To ease this problem, healthcare assistants are being increasingly used to undertake some of the more mundane tasks.

Audit

Intensive care audit is highly sophisticated and detailed. Dedicated staff are often required to assist with data collection which includes information on diagnoses, demographics, severity, resource use, and outcome. Methods such as severity scoring are being developed to adjust for case mix to enable comparisons within and between units. The establishment of the Intensive Care National Audit Research Centre (ICNARC) and Scottish Intensive Care Society Audit Group has been an important step in this respect. ICNARC has recently developed

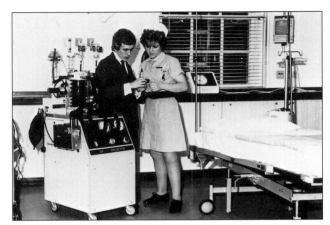

Mechanical ventilator, 1969

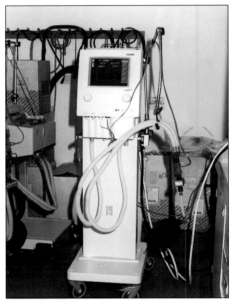

Mechanical ventilator, 1999

Role of other health careprofessionals in intensive care

Professional	Role
Physiotherapists	Prevent and treat chest problems, assist mobilisation, and prevent contractures in immobilised patients
Pharmacists	Advise on potential drug interactions and side effects, and drug dosing in patients with liver or renal dysfunction
Dietitians	Advise on nutritional requirements and feeds
Microbiologists	Advise on treatment and infection control
Medical physics technicians	Maintain equipment, including patient monitors, ventilators, haemofiltration machines, and blood gas analysers

Effective audit is essential for evaluating treatments in intensive care

a national case mix programme, to which many UK intensive care units subscribe.

Cost

Intensive care is expensive. The cost per bed day is £1000-£1800 with salaries accounting for over 60%, pharmacy for 10%, and disposables for a further 10%. The current contracting process has found it difficult to account for intensive care, partly because it does not have multidisciplinary specialty status and is therefore extremely difficult to isolate from the structure of the "finished consultant episode." This has been partially resolved by the development of the augmented care period (except in Scotland), defined by 12 data items which include information about the duration and intensity of care. It is intended that this will become part of hospital administration systems and improve the process of contracting for intensive care services. This is essential for budgetary health and the development of intensive care as an independent multidisciplinary specialty. In the United Kingdom, in parallel with many other countries, specialty status is in the process of being officially accorded.

The intensive care budget often falls within a directorate such as anaesthesia or theatres, although large units may have a separate budget. Units now have a business manager, who may be employed specifically for this role or, more commonly, be a senior nurse. This is a daunting task. Severe constraints are often rigorously applied by the hospital management leading to bed closures and an inability to replace ageing equipment.

Caring for relatives and patients

The intensive care environment can be extremely distressing for both relatives and conscious patients. The high mortality and morbidity of patients requires considerable psychological and emotional support. This is provided by the medical and nursing staff often in conjunction with chaplains and professional and lay counsellors. Such support is difficult and time consuming and requires the involvement of senior staff.

Many relatives and close friends wish to be close to critically ill patients at all times. Visiting times are usually flexible and many units have a dedicated visitors' sitting room with basic amenities such as a kitchenette, television, and toilet facilities. On site overnight accommodation can often be provided.

Summary

Few large scale studies exist of intensive care. This is partly because the patient population is heterogeneous and difficult to investigate. Although clinical management varies according to local need and facilities and the views of medical and nursing staff, similar philosophies are generally adopted.

Underprovision of intensive care is likely to dominate policy decisions in the near future. Intensive care will probably have an increasingly important role as the general population ages and the expectation for health care and the complexity of surgery increases.

The picture of the patient with polio was provided by *Danske Fysioterpeuter* (Danish journal of physiotherapy). We thank Radiometer UK and St George's Hospital archivist for help.

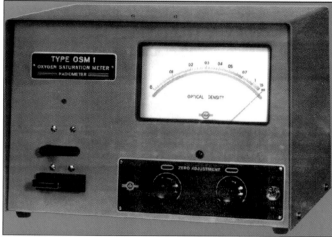

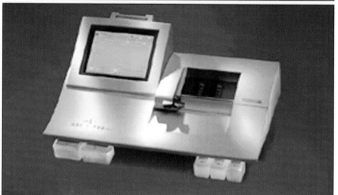

Blood gas analysers, 1964 and 1999: technological developments have improved patient care but added to the cost

---

Key points
- Organisation of intensive care units in the United Kingdom varies widely
- Clinical managements strategies are determined by local need, facilities, and staff
- Lack of large scale studies has hampered consensus on treatment
- Underprovision of intensive care is likely to dominate policy decisions in near future

---

2 Criteria for admission

Gary Smith, Mick Nielsen

Intensive care has been defined as "a service for patients with potentially recoverable conditions who can benefit from more detailed observation and invasive treatment than can safely be provided in general wards or high dependency areas." It is usually reserved for patients with potential or established organ failure. The most commonly supported organ is the lung, but facilities should also exist for the diagnosis, prevention, and treatment of other organ dysfunction.

Who to admit

Intensive care is appropriate for patients requiring or likely to require advanced respiratory support, patients requiring support of two or more organ systems, and patients with chronic impairment of one or more organ systems who also require support for an acute reversible failure of another organ. Early referral is particularly important. If referral is delayed until the patient's life is clearly at risk, the chances of full recovery are jeopardised.

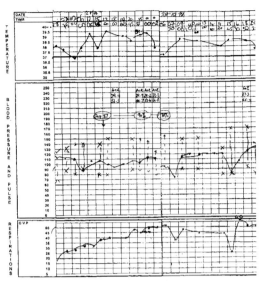

Ward observation chart showing serious physiological deterioration

---

Categories of organ system monitoring and support
(Adapted from *Guidelines on admission to and discharge from intensive care and high dependency units.* London: Department of Health, 1996.)

Advanced respiratory support
● Mechanical ventilatory support (excluding mask continuous positive airway pressure (CPAP) or non-invasive (eg, mask) ventilation)
● Possibility of a sudden, precipitous deterioration in respiratory function requiring immediate endotracheal intubation and mechanical ventilation

Basic respiratory monitoring and support
● Need for more than 50% oxygen
● Possibility of progressive deterioration to needing advanced respiratory support
● Need for physiotherapy to clear secretions at least two hourly
● Patients recently extubated after prolonged intubation and mechanical ventilation
● Need for mask continuous positive airway pressure or non-invasive ventilation
● Patients who are intubated to protect the airway but require no ventilatory support and who are otherwise stable

Circulatory support
● Need for vasoactive drugs to support arterial pressure or cardiac output
● Support for circulatory instability due to hypovolaemia from any cause which is unresponsive to modest volume replacement (including post-surgical or gastrointestinal haemorrhage or haemorrhage related to a coagulopathy)
● Patients resuscitated after cardiac arrest where intensive or high dependency care is considered clinically appropriate
● Intra-aortic balloon pumping

Neurological monitoring and support
● Central nervous system depression, from whatever cause, sufficient to prejudice the airway and protective reflexes
● Invasive neurological monitoring

Renal support
● Need for acute renal replacement therapy (haemodialysis, haemofiltration, or haemodiafiltration)

As with any other treatment, the decision to admit a patient to an intensive care unit should be based on the concept of potential benefit. Patients who are too well to benefit or those with no hope of recovering to an acceptable quality of life should not be admitted. Age by itself should not be a barrier to admission to intensive care, but doctors should recognise that increasing age is associated with diminishing physiological reserve and an increasing chance of serious coexisting disease. It is important to respect patient autonomy, and patients should not be admitted to intensive care if they have a stated or written desire not to receive intensive care—for example, in an advanced directive.

Severity of illness scoring systems such as the acute physiology and chronic health evaluation (APACHE) and simplified acute physiology score (SAPS) estimate hospital mortality for groups of patients. They cannot be used to predict which patients will benefit from intensive care as they are not sufficiently accurate and have not been validated for use before admission.

Factors to be considered when assessing suitability for admission to intensive care

● Diagnosis
● Severity of illness
● Age
● Coexisting disease
● Physiological reserve
● Prognosis
● Availability of suitable treatment
● Response to treatment to date
● Recent cardiopulmonary arrest
● Anticipated quality of life
● The patient's wishes

When to admit

Patients should be admitted to intensive care before their condition reaches a point from which recovery is impossible. Clear criteria may help to identify those at risk and to trigger a call for help from intensive care staff. Early referral improves the chances of recovery, reduces the potential for organ dysfunction (both extent and number), may reduce length of stay in intensive care and hospital, and may reduce the costs of intensive care. Patients should be referred by the most senior member of staff responsible for the patient—that is, a consultant. The decision should be delegated to trainee doctors only if clear guidelines exist on admission. Once patients are stabilised they should be transferred to the intensive care unit by experienced intensive care staff with appropriate transfer equipment.

Initial treatment

In critical illness the need to support the patient's vital functions may, at least initially, take priority over establishing a precise diagnosis. For example, patients with life threatening shock need immediate treatment rather than diagnosis of the cause as the principles of management are the same whether shock results from a massive myocardial infarction or a gastrointestinal bleed. Similarly, although the actual management may differ, the principles of treating other life threatening organ failures—for example, respiratory failure or coma—do not depend on precise diagnosis.

Respiratory support

All seriously ill patients without pre-existing lung disease should receive supplementary oxygen at sufficient concentration to maintain arterial oxygen tension ≥8 kPa or oxygen saturation of at least 90%. In patients with depressed ventilation (type II respiratory failure) oxygen will correct the hypoxaemia but not the hypercapnia. Care is required when monitoring such patients by pulse oximetry as it does not detect hypercapnia.

A few patients with severe chronic lung disease are dependent on hypoxic respiratory drive, and oxygen may depress ventilation. Nevertheless, life threatening hypoxaemia must be avoided, and if this requires concentrations of oxygen that exacerbate hypercapnia the patient will probably need mechanical ventilation.

Any patient who requires an inspired oxygen concentration of 50% or more should ideally be managed at least on a high dependency unit. Referral to intensive care should not be based solely on the need for endotracheal intubation or mechanical ventilation as early and aggressive intervention, high intensity nursing, and careful monitoring may prevent further deterioration. Endotracheal intubation can maintain a patent airway and protect it from contamination by foreign material such as regurgitated or vomited gastric contents or blood. Putting the patient in the recovery position with the head down helps protect the airway while awaiting the necessary expertise for intubation. Similarly, simple adjuncts such as an oropharyngeal airway may help to maintain airway patency, although it does not give the protection of an endotracheal tube.

Breathlessness and respiratory difficulty are common in acutely ill patients. Most will not need mechanical ventilation, but those that do require ventilation need to be identified as early as possible and certainly before they deteriorate to the point of respiratory arrest. The results of blood gas analysis alone are rarely sufficient to determine the need for mechanical ventilation. Several other factors have to be taken into consideration:

Criteria for calling intensive care staff to adult patients
(Adapted from McQuillan et al *BMJ* 1998;316:1853-8.)

- Threatened airway
- All respiratory arrests
- Respiratory rate ≥40 or ≤8 breaths/min
- Oxygen saturation <90% on ≥50% oxygen
- All cardiac arrests
- Pulse rate <40 or >140 beats/min
- Systolic blood pressure <90 mm Hg
- Sudden fall in level of consciousness (fall in Glasgow coma score >2 points)
- Repeated or prolonged seizures
- Rising arterial carbon dioxide tension with respiratory acidosis
- Any patient giving cause for concern

Basic monitoring requirements for seriously ill patients

- Heart rate
- Blood pressure
- Respiratory rate
- Pulse oximetry
- Hourly urine output
- Temperature
- Blood gases

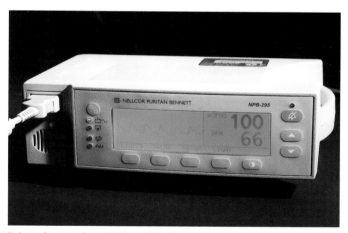

Pulse oximeters give no information about presence or absence of hypercapnia

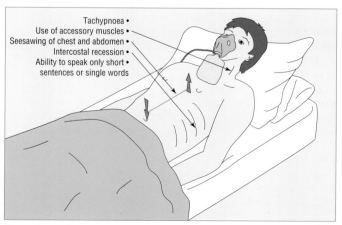

Signs of excessive respiratory work

Degree of respiratory work—A patient with normal blood gas tensions who is working to the point of exhaustion is more likely to need ventilating than one with abnormal tensions who is alert, oriented, talking in full sentences, and not working excessively.

Likely normal blood gas tensions for that patient—Some patients with severe chronic lung disease will lead surprisingly normal lives with blood gas tensions which would suggest the need for ventilation in someone previously fit.

Likely course of disease—If imminent improvement is likely ventilation can be deferred, although such patients need close observation and frequent blood gas analysis.

Adequacy of circulation—A patient with established or threatened circulatory failure as well as respiratory failure should be ventilated early in order to gain control of at least one major determinant of tissue oxygen delivery.

Circulatory support

Shock represents a failure of tissue perfusion. As such, it is primarily a failure of blood flow and not blood pressure. Nevertheless, an adequate arterial pressure is essential for perfusion of major organs and glomerular filtration, particularly in elderly or hypertensive patients, and for sustaining flow through any areas of critical narrowing in the coronary and cerebral vessels. A normal blood pressure does not exclude shock since pressure may be maintained at the expense of flow by vasoconstriction. Conversely, a high cardiac output (for example, in sepsis) does not preclude regional hypoperfusion associated with systemic vasodilatation, hypotension, and maldistribution.

Shock may be caused by hypovolaemia (relative or actual), myocardial dysfunction, microcirculatory abnormalities, or a combination of these factors. To identify shock it is important to recognise the signs of failing tissue perfusion.

All shocked patients should receive supplementary oxygen. Thereafter, the principles of management are to ensure an adequate circulating volume and then, if necessary, to give vasoactive drugs (for example, inotropes, vasopressors, vasodilators) to optimise cardiac output (and hence tissue oxygen delivery) and correct hypotension. Most patients will need intravenous fluid whatever the underlying disease. Central venous pressure may guide volume replacement and should be considered in patients who fail to improve despite an initial litre of intravenous fluid or sooner in patients with known or suspected myocardial dysfunction. Any patients needing more than modest fluid replacement or who require vasoactive drugs to support arterial pressure or cardiac output should be referred for high dependency or intensive care.

Neurological support

Neurological failure may occur after head injury, poisoning, cerebral vascular accident, infections of the nervous system (meningitis or encephalitis), cardiac arrest, or as a feature of metabolic encephalopathy (such as liver failure). The sequelae of neurological impairment may lead to the patient requiring intensive care. For instance, loss of consciousness may lead to obstruction of airways, loss of protective airway reflexes, and disordered ventilation that requires intubation or tracheostomy and mechanical ventilation.

Neurological disease may also cause prolonged or recurrent seizures or a rise in intracranial pressure. Patients who need potent anaesthetic drugs such as thiopentone or propofol to treat seizures that are resistant to conventional anticonvulsants, or monitoring of intracranial pressure and cerebral perfusion pressure must be referred to a high dependency or intensive care unit. Patients with neuromuscular disease (for example,

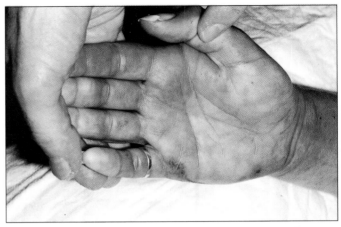

Peripheral cyanosis and poor capillary refill indicate failing circulation

Signs suggestive of failing tissue perfusion

- Tachycardia
- Confusion or diminished conscious level
- Poor peripheral perfusion (cool, cyanosed extremities, poor capillary refill, poor peripheral pulses)
- Poor urine output (< 0.5 ml/kg/h)
- Metabolic acidosis
- Increased blood lactate concentration

Normal blood pressure does not exclude shock

Neurological considerations in referral to intensive care

- Airway obstruction
- Absent gag or cough reflex
- Measurement of intracranial pressure and cerebral perfusion pressure
- Raised intracranial pressure requiring treatment
- Prolonged or recurrent seizures which are resistant to conventional anticonvulsants
- Hypoxaemia
- Hypercapnia or hypocapnia

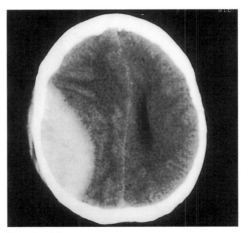

Extradural haematoma

Guillain-Barré syndrome, myasthenia gravis) may require admission to intensive care for intubation or ventilation because of respiratory failure, loss of airway reflexes, or aspiration.

Renal support

Renal failure is a common complication of acute illness or trauma and the need for renal replacement therapy (haemofiltration, haemodialysis, or their variants) may be a factor when considering referral to intensive or high dependency care. The need for renal replacement therapy is determined by assessment of urine volume, fluid balance, renal concentrating power (for example, urine:plasma osmolality ratio and urinary sodium concentration), acid-base balance, and the rate of rise of plasma urea, creatinine, and potassium concentrations. In ill patients hourly recording of urine output on the ward may give an early indication of a developing renal problem; prompt treatment, including aggressive circulatory resuscitation, may prevent this from progressing to established renal failure.

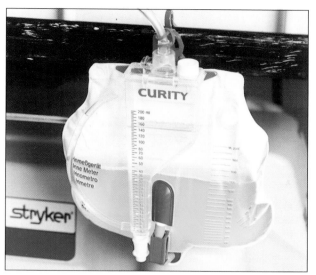

Measurement of urine output is important to detect renal problems promptly

Indications for considering renal replacement therapy
- Oliguria (<0.5ml/kg/h)
- Life threatening hyperkalaemia (>6 mmol/l) resistant to drug treatment
- Rising plasma concentrations of urea or creatinine, or both
- Severe metabolic acidosis
- Symptoms related to uraemia (for example, pericarditis, encephalopathy)

3 Organ dysfunction

Timothy W Evans, Mark Smithies

Most illness and death in patients in intensive care is caused by the consequences of sepsis and systemic inflammation. These conditions are responsible for an estimated 100 000 deaths a year in the United States alone. The systemic inflammatory response syndrome (SIRS) produces a clinical reaction that is indistinguishable from sepsis in the absence of an infecting organism

.

> **Understanding the pathogenesis of multiple organ failure is the key to reducing the unacceptably high mortality associated with sepsis**

Definitions of systemic inflammatory response syndrome (SIRS), sepsis, septic shock, and multiple organ dysfunction syndrome (American College of Chest Physicians, 1992)

Systemic inflammatory response syndrome
Two or more of the following clinical signs of systemic response to endothelial inflammation:
- Temperature $>38°C$ or $<36°C$
- Heart rate >90 beats/min
- Tachypnoea (respiratory rate >20 breaths/min or hyperventilation ($Paco_2 < 4.25$ kPa))
- White blood cell count $>12 \times 10^9/l$ or $<4 \times 10^9/l$ or the presence of more than 10% immature neutrophils
  In the setting (or strong suspicion) of a known cause of endothelial inflammation such as:
- Infection (bacteria, viruses, fungi, parasites, yeasts, or other organisms)
- Pancreatitis
- Ischaemia
- Multiple trauma and tissue injury
- Haemorrhagic shock
- Immune mediated organ injury
- Absence of any other known cause for such clinical abnormalities

Sepsis
Systemic response to infection manifested by two or more of the following:
- Temperature $>38°C$ or $<36°C$
- Raised heart rate $>90/min$
- Tachypnoea (respiratory rate >20 breaths/min or hyperventilation ($Paco_2 < 4.25$ kPa))
- White blood cell count $>12 \times 10^9/l$ or $<4 \times 10^9/l$ or the presence of more than 10% immature neutrophils

Septic shock
Sepsis induced hypotension (systolic blood pressure <90 mm Hg or a reduction of ≥ 40 mm Hg from baseline) despite adequate fluid resuscitation

Multiple organ dysfunction syndrome
Presence of altered organ function in an acutely ill patient such that homoeostasis cannot be maintained without intervention

---

Pathogenesis

Systemic sepsis may complicate an obvious primary infection such as community acquired pneumonia or a ruptured abdominal viscus. Frequently, however, an infective source cannot be identified and the type of organism cultured may provide no clue to its anatomical origin.

Infections that complicate critical illness may arise from the gastrointestinal tract. This region is particularly sensitive to poor perfusion, which may lead to increased bowel permeability and translocation of organisms and endotoxin from the lumen of the gastrointestinal tract into the portal venous and lymphatic circulations. The subsequent release of cytokines and other inflammatory mediators by hepatic Kupffer cells and circulating monocytes may then initiate a sequence of events that culminates in the clinical signs of sepsis and multiple organ failure.

Scientific background

The movement of oxygen, the regulation of its distribution between and within tissues, and the monitoring of cellular metabolism are all important in the clinical management of critically ill patients. Patients with sepsis or the systemic inflammatory response syndrome have a haemodynamic disturbance characterised by a raised cardiac output and reduced systemic vascular resistance. Although delivery of oxygen may be maintained or even increased by pharmacological means, most patients have poor peripheral uptake of oxygen.

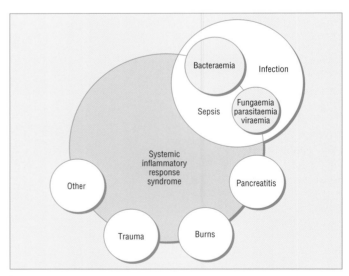

Relation between infection, sepsis, and systemic inflammatory response syndrome

> **Multiple organ failure may result from poor distribution of blood flow or a failure of cells to use oxygen because of the inflammatory process**

The cause of this phenomenon remains unclear. However, sepsis and systemic inflammatory response syndrome are associated with damage to the vascular endothelium, which normally produces vasoactive substances that regulate microvascular blood flow to ensure that all organs are adequately oxygenated. The microcirculation may therefore be disrupted. In addition, inflammatory mediators may modulate directly the intracellular mechanisms that regulate use of oxygen, including mitochondrial function. These two factors mean that patients with sepsis or the systemic inflammatory response syndrome commonly develop multiple organ failure, to which many succumb. Nevertheless, not all patients at risk of developing sepsis and multiple organ failure do so, and individual susceptibility varies widely.

Each patient's clinical response to the activation of inflammatory cascades may be determined by abnormalities of gene transcription and regulation that modulate the release of vasoactive substances such as nitric oxide, endothelins, and cyclo-oxygenase products (thromboxanes, prostaglandins, etc). Additionally, changes in the effectiveness of endogenous defence systems such as cellular antioxidant protection, repair, and apoptosis may be relevant in determining outcome. In any event, the clinical result of these perturbations is tissue hypoxia.

Detection of tissue hypoxia

The clinical signs of tissue hypoxia are largely non-specific. However, increased respiratory rate, peripheries that are either warm and vasodilated or cold and vasoconstricted, poor urine output, and mental dullness may indicate organ dysfunction and should prompt a search for reversible causes. The following biochemical and physiological measurements may be helpful.

Metabolic acidosis
A low arterial pH and high blood lactate concentration may be important. Anaerobic production of lactate may occur secondary to global hypoxia (for example, cardiorespiratory failure or septic shock) or focal hypoxia (for example, infarcted bowel) or through non-hypoxic causes (for example, delayed lactate clearance, accelerated aerobic glycolysis, or dysfunction of pyruvate dehydrogenase). A wide arterial-mixed venous carbon dioxide pressure gradient (>1 kPa) has been shown to be relatively insensitive as a marker of anaerobic tissue metabolism.

Oxygen extraction ratio
The uptake of oxygen by tissues (Vo_2) is normally independent of oxygen delivery (Do_2). If delivery fails the oxygen extraction ratio (Vo_2:Do_2) rises to maintain a constant rate of uptake and fulfil tissue demand. The compensatory mechanisms fail only at very low oxygen delivery levels (termed Do_{2Crit}), when extraction starts to fall and become dependent on delivery. However, patients with sepsis or the systemic inflammatory response syndrome have a low oxygen extraction ratio, indicating poor tissue uptake or use. Changes in oxygen delivery and uptake relations have been used to identify occult tissue hypoxia and predict outcome since those who survive septic shock tend to achieve normal oxygen extraction levels.

Increasing oxygen delivery in these patients should produce a corresponding increase in uptake. However, in practice this is difficult to ascertain because of problems in measurement and the need for tissue oxygen demand to remain constant.

Recent randomised clinical trials have also indicated that patients receiving treatment designed to increase oxygen delivery and uptake may have greater mortality than controls. A

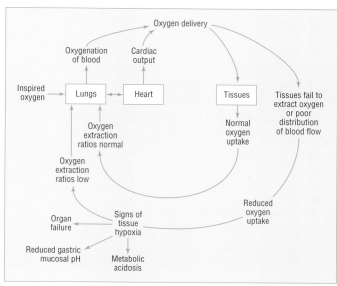

Generation of tissue hypoxia. Oxygen delivery is the product of arterial oxygen content and cardiac output. In systemic inflammatory response syndrome or sepsis blood flow is poorly distributed or tissues fail to use oxygen. Signs of tissue hypoperfusion are apparent and mixed venous oxygen saturation may be increased

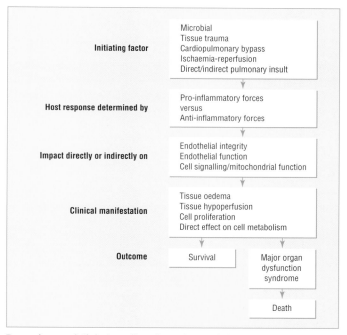

Determinants of clinical manifestations of systemic inflammatory response syndrome and sepsis

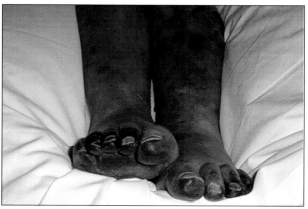

Poor peripheral perfusion

high mixed venous oxygen saturation, measured through a pulmonary artery catheter, indirectly indicates a low oxygen extraction ratio.

Gastric mucosal pH (pHi)

Gastric mucosal pH can be measured using a tonometer, originally a saline filled balloon placed in the gastric lumen. If the arterial bicarbonate concentration is known, the carbon dioxide tension in the saline samples withdrawn from the balloon can be used to calculate the pH. Several studies have found that a falling or persistently low gastric mucosal pH is associated with poor prognosis in critically ill patients. However, whether gastric mucosal pH truly provides evidence of gastric mucosal hypoxia remains uncertain. Tonometers are now becoming semiautomated and use air instead of saline. Measurement of gastric-arterial carbon dioxide tension or gastric-end-tidal carbon dioxide tension differences has been suggested instead of gastric mucosal pH.

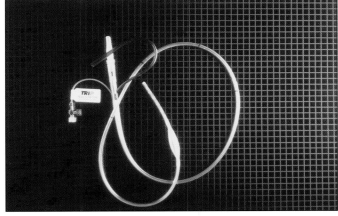

Gastric tonometer

Injury to individual organs

Lung injury

About 35% of patients with sepsis develop mild to moderate acute lung injury and a quarter have fully developed acute respiratory distress syndrome. Affected patients have increased pulmonary vascular permeability, which leads to alveolar oedema and refractory hypoxaemia. Lung injury rarely occurs in isolation. It is usually the pulmonary manifestation of a pan-endothelial insult with inflammatory vascular dysfunction. The annual incidence of acute respiratory distress syndrome is about 6 cases per 100 000 population. Data on incidence and outcome of acute lung injury, which was defined relatively recently, are sparse.

Acute lung injury and the acute respiratory distress syndrome may have different causes as the acute respiratory distress syndrome is partly determined by the nature of the underlying or precipitating condition. Moreover, the precipitating condition and coexisting multiple organ failure dictate outcome. The increased permeability of the alveolar capillary membrane in these conditions suggests that lowering filling pressures by aggressive diuresis or early ultrafiltration may improve oxygenation. However, any concomitant decrease in cardiac output can result in an overall fall in oxygen delivery and may prejudice the perfusion of other organs.

Cardiovascular injury

Myocardial dysfunction also complicates sepsis and the systemic inflammatory response syndrome. Ventricular dilatation occurs in patients with septic shock, and the ejection fraction may be reduced to around 30% despite an overall rise in measured cardiac output. Patients who die tend to have had lower end diastolic volumes and less compliant ventricles during diastole than survivors. Normal volunteers given endotoxin also develop left ventricular dilatation during diastole, suggesting that cardiac function is greatly affected in septic shock. The cellular changes behind ventricular dilatation are unknown.

Systemic vascular resistance is also low in sepsis, possibly through overexpression of vasodilator substances such as nitric oxide and cyclo-oxygenase products in the vascular smooth muscle. The consequent loss of vasoregulation may result in poor distribution of perfusion and tissue hypoxia.

Optimisation of left ventricular filling pressure, inotropic support, and vasoconstrictors such as noradrenaline are all beneficial in septic shock. In addition, novel pressor agents such as nitric oxide synthase inhibitors have been advocated recently

Recommended diagnostic criteria for acute lung injury and acute respiratory distress syndrome

Criteria	Acute lung injury	Acute respiratory distress syndrome
Onset	Acute	Acute
Oxygenation*	$Pao_2/Fio_2 \leqslant 300$	$Pao_2/Fio_2 \leqslant 200$
Chest radiograph (frontal)	Bilateral infiltrates	Bilateral infiltrates
Pulmonary artery wedge pressure	$\leqslant 18$ mm Hg or no clinical evidence of raised left atrial pressure	$\leqslant 18$ mm Hg or no clinical evidence of raised left atrial pressure

*Oxygenation to be considered regardless of the positive end expiratory pressure. Pao_2 = arterial oxygen tension, Fio_2 = fraction of inspired oxygen.

Adapted from Bernard et al *Am J Respir Crit Care Med* 1994;149:818-24.

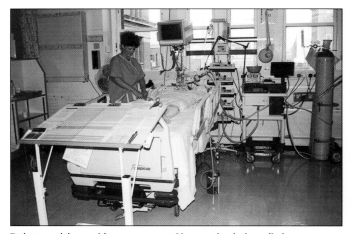

Patient receiving multisystem support. Note mechanical ventilation, vasopressor agent infusions, and nitric oxide cylinder for nitric oxide inhalation

for patients with refractory septic shock. Increased knowledge of the changes in vascular biology that characterise sepsis and the systemic inflammatory response syndrome may allow transient genetic manipulation of the expression of vasoactive mediators that control microvascular distribution of blood flow.

Renal failure

Acute renal failure is a common complication of sepsis and the systemic inflammatory response syndrome. This may reflect changes in the distribution of intrarenal blood flow between the cortex and medulla. The ability of patients to maintain intravascular homoeostasis may also be impaired. The early use of haemofiltration to correct fluid imbalance and (possibly) remove circulating inflammatory mediators has been advocated, but the benefits are unproved. It is essential to restore circulating volume and achieve an adequate blood pressure and cardiac output to prevent and treat acute renal failure.

Dysfunction of gastrointestinal tract

The bowel is particularly susceptible to ischaemic insults. Hypoperfusion of the gastrointestinal tract is thought to be important in the pathogenesis of multiple organ failure as outlined above. Hepatic dysfunction, possibly resulting from reduced blood flow relative to metabolic demand, is also common in critically ill patients. Maintaining adequate flow and perfusion pressure are the only proved treatments to correct these deficiencies. Inotropic drugs with dilator properties such as dopexamine may selectively enhance splanchnic perfusion and oxygenation. Nevertheless, well controlled trials of augmented oxygen transport (possibly guided by gastric tonometry) are needed to establish the role of the gastrointestinal tract in multiple organ failure.

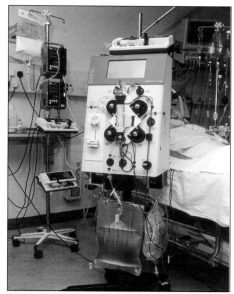

Benefits of early haemofiltration are unproved

Key points

- Organ dysfunction probably arises from abnormalities of microvascular control and cellular metabolism
- Susceptibility to the effects of inflammatory activation may be determined genetically
- The gastrointestinal tract seems to be the "motor" of sepsis
- New supportive and therapeutic interventions are emerging as understanding of sepsis increases

4 Respiratory support

Maire P Shelly, Peter Nightingale

Most patients admitted to intensive care require some form of respiratory support. This is usually because of hypoxaemia or ventilatory failure, or both. The support offered ranges from oxygen therapy by face mask, through non-invasive techniques such as continuous positive airways pressure, to full ventilatory support with endotracheal intubation.

Oxygen therapy

Oxygen is given to treat hypoxaemia. Patients should initially be given a high concentration. The amount can then be adjusted according to the results of pulse oximetry and arterial blood gas analysis. The dangers of reducing hypoxic drive have been overemphasised; hypoxaemia is more dangerous than hypercapnia. The theoretical dangers of oxygen toxicity are unimportant if the patient is hypoxaemic.

Oxygen is usually given by face mask, although nasal prongs or cannulas may be better tolerated. A fixed performance, high flow, air entrainment mask can provide a known fractional inspired oxygen concentration (Fio_2) within the range 0.24-0.60. The fractional inspired oxygen concentration is not known with the more common variable performance masks. The maximum concentration is 0.6 unless a reservoir bag is added to the mask.

Non-invasive respiratory support

If the patient remains hypoxaemic on high flow oxygen (15 l/min) continuous positive airways pressure (CPAP) may be used. The technique improves oxygenation by recruiting underventilated alveoli and so is most successful in clinical situations where alveoli are readily recruited, such as acute pulmonary oedema and postoperative atelectasis. It is also helpful in immunocompromised patients with pneumonia. As intubation is avoided the risks of nosocomial pneumonia are reduced. The continuous positive airways pressure mask often becomes uncomfortable and gastric distension may occur. Patients must therefore be cooperative, able to protect their airway, and have the strength to breathe spontaneously and cough effectively.

Non-invasive ventilation refers to ventilatory support without tracheal intubation. This can be used as a first step in patients who require some ventilatory support and who are not profoundly hypoxaemic. Ventilation through a nasal or face mask may avoid the need for intubation, especially in exacerbations of chronic obstructive airways disease. Some patients with chronic ventilatory failure rely on long term non-invasive ventilation. It may also have a place during weaning from conventional ventilation. External negative pressure ventilation, historically provided by an "iron lung," is now provided by a cuirass system.

Ventilatory support

Endotracheal intubation and ventilation is the next step in the management of respiratory failure. Clinical symptoms and signs are generally more useful than arterial blood gas analysis or measurements of peak expiratory flow rate and vital capacity in deciding the need for intubation.. However, some findings

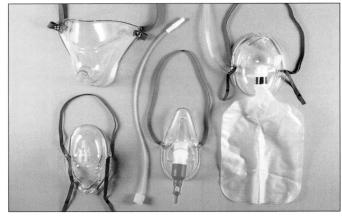
Oxygen masks and nasal cannula

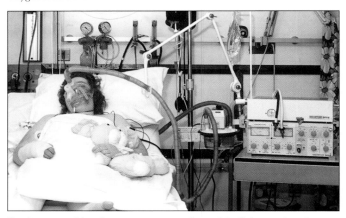
Continuous positive airways pressure requires a tight fitting mask and appropriate valve and breathing system

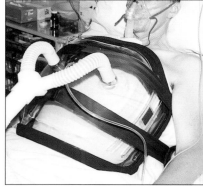
Hayek oscillator provides external negative pressure ventilation

---

Indications for intubation and ventilation

- Protect the airway—for example, facial trauma or burns, unconscious patient
- Treat profound hypoxaemia—for example, pneumonia, cardiogenic pulmonary oedema, acute respiratory distress syndrome
- Postoperative care—for example, after cardiothoracic surgery and other major, complicated, or prolonged surgery
- Allow removal of secretions—for example, myasthenia gravis, Guillain-Barré syndrome
- Rest exhausted patients—for example, severe asthma
- Avoid or control hypercapnia—for example, acute brain injury, hepatic coma, chronic obstructive airways disease

---

confirm the imminent need for ventilation. These include hypoxaemia in patients receiving maximum oxygen therapy ($Pao_2 < 8$ kPa, or $Sao_2 < 90\%$), hypercapnia with impairment of conscious level, and a falling vital capacity in patients with neuromuscular disorders.

Management of the airway

Endotracheal intubation can be extremely hazardous in critically ill patients with respiratory and often cardiovascular failure. Continuous monitoring, particularly of heart rate and blood pressure, is essential and resuscitation drugs must be immediately available.

Hypotension follows induction of anaesthesia because of the direct cardiovascular effects of the drugs given. Unconsciousness also reduces intrinsic sympathetic drive. Positive pressure ventilation reduces venous return to the heart and reduces cardiac output.

Tracheostomies are usually done electively when intubation is likely to be prolonged (over 14 days). They may also be done for the patient's comfort and to facilitate weaning from the ventilator. Tracheostomy is often done as a percutaneous procedure in intensive care. Complications of tracheostomy include misplacement or displacement of the tube, bleeding, infection, failure of the stoma to heal, and tracheal stenosis. However, because patients tolerate a tracheostomy much better than an orotracheal tube, sedation can usually be reduced, weaning is more rapid, and the stay in intensive care is reduced. A minitracheostomy may help with tracheal toilet in patients with copious secretions and poor cough effort.

Ventilator strategy

The choice of ventilatory mode and settings such as tidal volume, respiratory rate, positive end expiratory pressure (PEEP), and the ratio of inspiratory to expiratory time depends on the patient's illness. In asthma, for example, a prolonged expiratory phase may be required for lung deflation, whereas in patients with atelectasis or other forms of reduced lung volume the emphasis is towards recruiting alveoli with positive end expiratory pressure or a prolonged inspiratory phase.

Damage to lungs can be exacerbated by mechanical ventilation, possibly because of overdistension of alveoli and the repeated opening and collapse of distal airways. Some evidence exists for benefit from a lung protective ventilatory strategy using positive end expiratory pressure or prolonged inspiration to maintain alveolar volume, and limiting tidal volumes and peak airway pressures. This may result in increased arterial carbon dioxide pressure (permissive hypercapnia). Serial measurements of airway pressure and tidal volume allow lung compliance to be optimised. Compliance indicates alveolar recruitment, and reduces the risks of overdistension.

Methods of ventilation

No consensus exists on the best method of ventilation. In volume controlled methods the ventilator delivers a preset tidal volume. The inspiratory pressure depends on the resistance and compliance of the respiratory system. In pressure controlled ventilation the delivered pressure is preset. Tidal volume varies according to the resistance and compliance of the respiratory system. Pressure controlled ventilation has become popular for severe acute respiratory distress syndrome as part of the lung protective strategy. As well as limiting peak airway pressure, the distribution of gas may be improved within the lung. Pressure controlled ventilation is often used with a long inspiratory

Indicators of respiratory distress

- Tachypnoea, dyspnoea
- Sweating
- Tachycardia and bounding pulse
- Agitation, restlessness, diminished conscious level, unwilling to lie flat
- Use of accessory muscles, intercostal recession
- Abdominal paradox (abdomen moves inward during inspiration)
- Respiratory alternans (thoracic movement then abdominal movement)
- Cyanosis or pallor

Potential problems during intubation

- Hypotension
- Reduced intrinsic sympathetic drive
- Reduced cardiac output
- Severe hypoxaemia
- Regurgitation and aspiration of gastric contents
- Arrhythmias
- Electrolyte disturbances, especially hyperkalaemia after suxamethonium

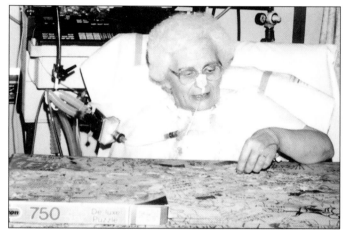

A tracheostomy is more comfortable than an orotracheal tube

Lung protective ventilation strategy

The strategy aims to maintain alveolar volume by
- Using lung recruitment manoeuvres and positive end expiratory pressure to maximise and maintain alveolar volume
- Avoiding alveolar overdistension by limiting tidal volume or airway pressure, or both

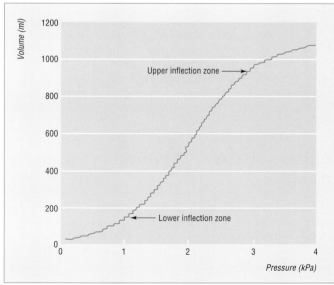

Pressure-volume curve showing upper and lower inflection points

phase (inverse ratio ventilation) to maintain adequate alveolar recruitment.

In high frequency techniques gas is delivered to the airway by oscillation or jet ventilation. The tidal volumes achieved are small but gas exchange still occurs. The role of high frequency techniques in respiratory support is not yet established.

Methods of ventilation that allow the patient to breathe spontaneously are thought to be advantageous. Modern ventilators have sensitive triggers and flow patterns that can adapt to the patient's needs, thus reducing the work of breathing. In synchronised intermittent mandatory ventilation a set number of breaths are delivered by the ventilator and the patient can breathe between these breaths. This method is often used during weaning, often with pressure support, by which the ventilator enhances the volume of each spontaneous breath up to a predetermined positive pressure. Biphasic airway pressure is similar to continuous positive airways pressure ventilation but pressure is set at two levels. The ventilator switches between the levels, thus augmenting alveolar ventilation.

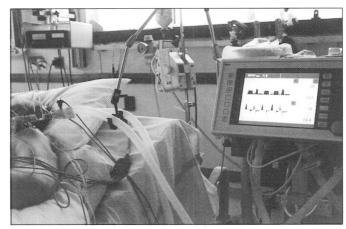

Biphasic airway pressure improves alveolar ventilation

Monitoring ventilatory therapy

Pulse oximetry and measurement of end tidal carbon dioxide concentration allow continuous monitoring of oxygenation and ventilation. End tidal carbon dioxide concentration is roughly equal to arterial carbon dioxide partial pressure in normal subjects but may differ widely in critically ill patients with ventilation-perfusion mismatch. Nevertheless, monitoring end tidal carbon dioxide may be useful in neurointensive care, when transferring critically ill patients, and for confirming tracheal intubation. Adequacy of ventilation should be confirmed regularly by arterial blood gas analysis. Tolerance to ventilation can be assessed using a simple scale.

Weaning from the ventilator

Several techniques are available for weaning. All are likely to fail unless the patient is well prepared. Clinical assessment is the most important issue in deciding when to wean a patient from the ventilator. The factors considered are similar to the indications for respiratory support. The patient should be adequately oxygenated ($Pao_2 > 8$ kPa with fractional inspired oxygen < 0.6); be able to maintain normocapnia; be able to meet the increased work of breathing; and be conscious and responsive. Weaning techniques allow the patient to breathe spontaneously for increasing periods or to gradually reduce the level of ventilatory support. Recently weaned patients should continue to be closely monitored for secondary deterioration. Patients are extubated after they are weaned from the ventilator and can breathe unaided. Patients also need to be able to protect their airway once it is no longer protected by an endotracheal tube. This means they must be alert, able to swallow without aspiration, and able to cough well enough to clear secretions.

Other aspects of respiratory support

Humidification

Inadequate humidification of inspired gases destroys the ciliated epithelium lining the upper airway. This stops secretions from being cleared from the lungs and increases the risk of infection. Piped medical oxygen and air are completely dry. The upper airway may not be able to supply enough heat and moisture to fully saturate them, especially when much of the upper airway is bypassed by tracheal intubation. Additional humidification is therefore necessary.

Ventilation assessment scale
- Tolerates ventilation
- Tolerates ventilation most of the time; some transient desaturation or coughing on manoeuvres such as tracheal suction, turning, etc
- Moderate desaturation on coughing or above manoeuvres that resolves spontaneously
- Severe or prolonged desaturation on coughing or above manoeuvres that requires intervention
- Intolerant of mechanical ventilation, requires manual intervention
- Paralysed

Preparation for weaning from the ventilator

Ensure
- Clear airway
- Adequate oxygenation
- Adequate carbon dioxide clearance

Control of
- Precipitating illness
- Fever and infection
- Pain
- Agitation
- Depression

Optimisation of
- Nutritional state
- Electrolytes (potassium, phosphate, magnesium)

Beware
- Excessive carbon dioxide production from overfeeding
- Sleep deprivation
- Acute left heart failure

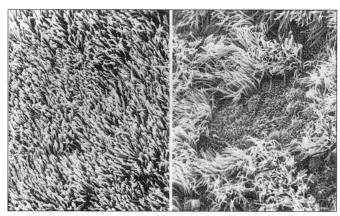

Inadequate humidification of inspired gases causes loss of tracheal and bronchial cilia (right), which reduces clearance of secretions from the lungs

Physiotherapy

Patients who are intubated cannot clear secretions effectively because of reduced conscious level, poor cough effort, and discomfort. Regular chest physiotherapy and tracheal suction are essential.

Position

Regular turning to avoid pressure sores also helps mobilise and clear secretions. Patients who are too unstable to be turned regularly may benefit from being nursed on special beds that allow some degree of rotation.

Patients with resistant hypoxaemia may benefit from being turned prone. The improved oxygenation probably results from normalisation of pleural pressure gradients within the lung.

Pharmacological adjuncts

Inhaled nitric oxide may improve oxygenation by dilating pulmonary vessels passing alongside ventilated alveoli. Although it is widely used, and often effective in increasing arterial oxygen tension in patients with acute respiratory distress syndrome, there is no evidence of improved survival. Nitric oxide remains unlicensed for this indication.

Steroids have a limited role in the acute management of ventilated patients except for treating the underlying disease—for example, asthma. However, there is evidence that they improve pulmonary function in the later, fibroproliferative, phase of acute respiratory distress syndrome.

Sedation

Ventilated patients generally require sedation to tolerate both ventilation and the presence of an endotracheal tube. The aim is for the patient to be comfortable at all times. In the past, ventilation could be controlled only if the patient was heavily sedated or even paralysed. Sophisticated ventilators now allow less sedation but patients still require analgesia for pain and relief of anxiety and distress.

Patients have individual needs and different indications for analgesia and sedation. Muscle relaxants are now used infrequently. Compassionate care and effective communication help patients, but drugs are often necessary to keep them comfortable.

Sedatives, however, have some adverse effects. The parent drug or active metabolites may accumulate because of renal failure and have prolonged action. There may also be circulatory effects—for example, hypotension. Tolerance sometimes occurs. Patients may develop withdrawal syndromes when the drug is stopped, while altered sleep patterns may produce sleep deprivation. Some patients develop ileus, which may impair feeding.

Because critically ill patients cannot usually say whether they are comfortable, anxiety, depression, and even pain may be difficult to assess. This assessment tends to be subjective and various scoring systems are used, most being based on the patient's response to different stimuli.

Conclusion

Many patients who would previously have died from respiratory failure now survive. Improved understanding and management of acute lung injury will hopefully lead to further improvements in survival. Appropriate treatment of hypoxia, and early referral to intensive care before complications arise, will also hopefully improve the outcome of critically ill patients.

The picture of cilia is reproduced with permission from Konrad F, Schiener R, Marx T, Georgieff M. *Intensive Care Medicine* 1995;21:482-9.

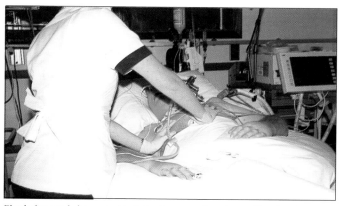

Physiotherapy is important to help clear secretions in ventilated patients

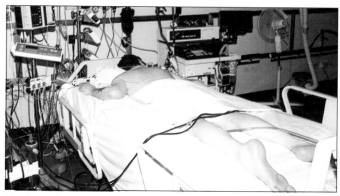

Nursing patients in prone position may help resistant hypoxaemia

---

Indications for analgesia and sedation

- Allow effective ventilation
- Reduce oxygen demand
- Provide analgesia
- Reduce anxiety
- Relieve distress
- Facilitate sleep
- Provide amnesia
- Reduce depression

Indications for muscle relaxants

- Allow intubation and other procedures
- Allow control of ventilation where respiratory drive is very high—for example, permissive hypercapnia
- Treat certain diseases—for example, tetanus
- Reduce oxygen demand while oxygenation is critical
- Control carbon dioxide pressure and prevent increases in intracranial pressure—for example, in head injury

---

Assessment of sedation

+3 Agitated and restless
+2 Awake and uncomfortable
+1 Aware but calm
0 Roused by voice
−1 Roused by touch
−2 Roused by painful stimuli
−3 Cannot be roused
A Natural sleep
P Paralysed

5   Circulatory support

C J Hinds, D Watson

Circulatory support is required not only for hypotension or shock but also to prevent complications in patients at risk of organ failure. Shock can be defined as "acute circulatory failure with inadequate or inappropriately distributed tissue perfusion resulting in generalised cellular hypoxia." It is a life threatening medical emergency.

Tissue perfusion may be jeopardised by cardiogenic, obstructive, hypovolaemic, or distributive shock. These factors often combine. For example, in sepsis and anaphylaxis, vascular dilatation and sequestration in venous capacitance vessels lead to relative hypovolaemia, which is compounded by true hypovolaemia due to fluid losses through increased microvascular permeability.

If abnormalities of tissue perfusion are allowed to persist, the function of vital organs will be impaired. The subsequent reperfusion will exacerbate organ dysfunction and, in severe cases, may culminate in multiple organ failure. Early recognition of patients who are shocked and immediate provision of effective circulatory support is therefore essential. Such support is usually best provided in an intensive care unit or high dependency area.

Cardiovascular monitoring

Blood pressure
Patients with a low cardiac output can sometimes maintain a reasonable blood pressure by vasoconstriction, while vasodilated patients may be hypotensive despite a high cardiac output. Blood pressure must always be assessed in relation to the patient's normal value. Percutaneous placement of an intra-arterial cannula allows continuous monitoring of blood pressure and repeated sampling of blood for gas and acid-base analysis. This is essential when rapid haemodynamic changes are anticipated—for example, when administering inotropic or vasoactive drugs.

Central venous pressure
Measurement of pressure within a large intrathoracic vein is a simple method of assessing circulating volume and myocardial function. However, the absolute value is often unhelpful, except in extreme cases of hypovolaemia, fluid overload, or heart failure. Correct interpretation requires assessment of the change in central venous pressure in response to a fluid challenge in conjunction with alterations in other monitored variables (such as heart rate, blood pressure, urine flow) and clinical signs (such as skin colour, peripheral temperature, and perfusion).

Pulmonary artery catheterisation
Catheterisation of the pulmonary artery with a balloon flotation catheter allows measurement of the filling pressure of the left ventricle (pulmonary artery occlusion pressure). As with central venous pressure, correct interpretation requires assessment of changes in pressure in response to treatment together with alterations in clinical signs and other monitored variables. Most patients who require pulmonary artery catheters should have their cardiac output measured (by a thermodilution technique.)

Pulmonary artery catheters can help establish the nature of the haemodynamic problem, optimise cardiac output while minimising the risk of pulmonary oedema, and allow the

Types of shock
- Cardiogenic shock: caused by "pump failure"—for example acute myocardial infarction
- Obstructive shock: caused by mechanical impediment to forward flow—for example, pulmonary embolus, cardiac tamponade
- Hypovolaemic shock: caused by loss of circulating volume. These losses may be exogenous (haemorrhage, burns) or endogenous (through leaks in the microcirculation or into body cavities as occurs in intestinal obstruction)
- Distributive shock: caused by abnormalities of the peripheral circulation—for example, sepsis and anaphylaxis

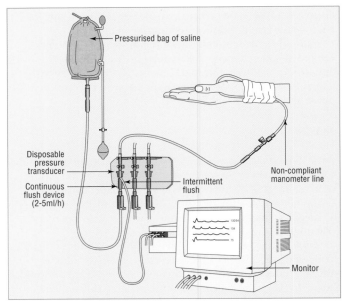

Continuous monitoring of blood pressure. A cannula placed percutaneously in an artery is connected to a pressure transducer through a fluid filled non-compliant manometer line incorporating a continuous and intermittent flush device. Adapted from Hinds CJ, Watson D. *Intensive care: a concise textbook.* WB Saunders, 1996.

Indications for pulmonary artery catheterisation
- Shock—unresponsive to simple measures or diagnostic uncertainty. To guide administration of fluid, inotropes, and vasopressors
- Haemodynamic instability when diagnosis unclear
- Major trauma—to guide volume replacement and haemodynamic support in severe cases
- Myocardial infarction—haemodynamic instability, unresponsive to initial therapy. To differentiate hypovolaemia from cardiogenic shock
- Pulmonary oedema—to differentiate cardiogenic from non-cardiogenic oedema. To guide haemodynamic support in cardiac failure and acute respiratory distress syndrome
- Chronic obstructive airways disease—patients with cardiac failure, to exclude reversible causes of difficulty in weaning from mechanical ventilation
- High risk surgical patients
- Cardiac surgery—selected cases only
- Pulmonary embolism—to assist in diagnosis and assess severity. To guide haemodynamic support
- Pre-eclampsia with hypertension, pulmonary oedema, and oliguria

rational use of inotropic and vasoactive drugs. Clinical haemodynamic assessment is often inaccurate. Pulmonary artery catheterisation improves diagnostic accuracy and provides information which often prompts changes in treatment. Nevertheless, its influence on outcome remains uncertain. Studies have suggested that the use of the catheters may be associated with a worse outcome. This may be due to the treatments used in response to the measurements obtained or inexperience with use of these catheters and interpretation of the data rather than to complications of the catheter.

Non-invasive techniques for assessing cardiac function

The most useful non-invasive technique for determining cardiac output and myocardial function is Doppler ultrasonography. A probe is passed into the oesophagus to continuously monitor velocity waveforms from the descending aorta. It is particularly valuable for perioperative optimisation of the circulating volume and cardiac performance.

Assessment of tissue perfusion

Clinical—Evaluate skin colour and temperature, capillary refill, pulse volume, and sweating.

Core–peripheral temperature gradient—An increase in the difference between central and peripheral temperature usually indicates hypovolaemia but is not a reliable guide to cardiac output or peripheral resistance

Urine output—A significant fall in renal perfusion is associated with oliguria which, if allowed to persist, may progress to acute tubular necrosis

Metabolic acidosis with raised blood lactate concentration may suggest that tissue perfusion is sufficiently compromised to cause cellular hypoxia, anaerobic glycolysis, and production of lactic acid. However, in many critically ill patients, especially those with sepsis, lactic acidosis is caused by metabolic disorders unrelated to tissue hypoxia and may be exacerbated by reduced clearance due to hepatic or renal dysfunction.

Gastric tonometry—The earliest compensatory response to hypovolaemia or a low cardiac output, and the last to resolve after resuscitation, is splanchnic vasoconstriction. In sepsis, gut mucosal ischaemia may be precipitated by disturbed microcirculatory flow combined with increased oxygen requirements. Mucosal acidosis is therefore an early sign of "compensated" shock. Changes in intramucosal pH or partial pressure of carbon dioxide have been suggested as a guide to the adequacy of resuscitation, although the clinical value of this technique remains uncertain.

Treatment of circulatory insufficiency

In all cases the objective is to restore oxygen delivery to the tissues while correcting the underlying cause (for example, surgical intervention to arrest haemorrhage or eradicate infection). Speed is essential. Delays in making the diagnosis and initiating treatment, as well as suboptimal resuscitation, contribute to the development of peripheral vascular failure and irreversible defects in oxygen use which can culminate in vital organ dysfunction.

Respiratory support

The first priority is to secure the airway and, if necessary, provide mechanical ventilation. Because mechanical ventilation abolishes or minimises the work of breathing, reduces oxygen consumption, and improves oxygenation, early respiratory support benefits patients with severe shock and those with cardiogenic shock complicated by pulmonary oedema.

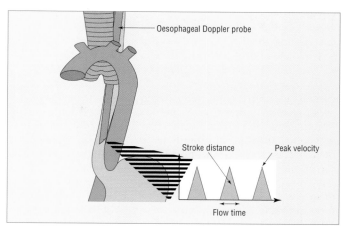

Oesophageal Doppler probe continuously measures velocity waveforms from the descending thoracic aorta. With a nomogram stroke distance (area under waveform) provides an estimate of stroke volume. Acceleration and peak velocity indicate myocardial performance while flow time is related to circulating volume and peripheral resistance

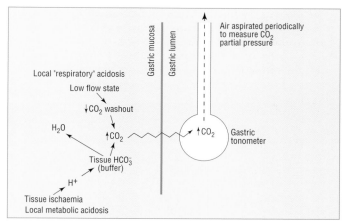

Gastric tonometry. Equilibration of carbon dioxide partial pressure between mucosa and balloon takes up to 30 minutes. Low flow states and tissue ischaemia are associated with a rise in carbon dioxide partial pressure

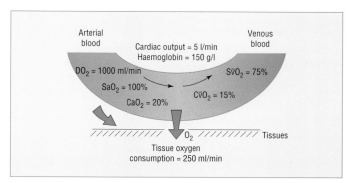

Oxygen delivery (the amount delivered to tissues per unit time) depends on the volume of blood flowing through the microcirculation (cardiac output) and the amount of oxygen the blood contains (arterial oxygen content (CaO_2)). Oxygen delivery (DO_2)=cardiac output×(haemoglobin concentration×oxygen saturation (SaO_2)×1.34). In normal adults it is roughly 1000 ml/min, of which 250 ml is taken up by tissues. Mixed venous blood is thus 75% saturated with oxygen. $C\bar{v}O_2$= mixed venous oxygen content, $S\bar{v}O_2$=mixed venous oxygen saturation

Patients with compromised circulatory function should always receive supplemental oxygen

Cardiovascular support

Tissue blood flow must be restored by achieving and maintaining an adequate cardiac output and by ensuring that systemic blood pressure is sufficient to maintain perfusion of vital organs. Traditionally, a mean arterial pressure of 60 mm Hg (or systolic blood pressure of 80 mm Hg) has been considered sufficient, but some evidence suggests that a mean pressure of 80 mm Hg may be more appropriate. Some people contend that the patient's normal blood pressure should be targeted. Circulatory support therefore involves manipulation of the three determinants of stroke volume (preload, myocardial contractility and afterload) as well as the heart rate.

Preload and volume replacement

Preload optimisation is the most efficient way of increasing cardiac output and is a prerequisite for restoring tissue perfusion. Controversy continues about whether colloids or crystalloids are preferable. The circulating volume must be replaced within minutes since rapid restoration of cardiac output and tissue perfusion pressure reduces the chances of serious organ damage, particularly acute renal failure.

As well as being fundamental to the management of hypovolaemic shock, replacement of the circulating volume is important in managing patients with impaired tissue perfusion due to cardiogenic, distributive, and obstructive causes. Adequate perioperative volume replacement also reduces morbidity and mortality in high risk surgical patients.

Inotropic and vasoactive agents

Before cardiac output and perfusion pressure are restored with drugs, abnormalities that might impair cardiac performance or vascular responsiveness—hypoxia, hypercalcaemia, and the effects of drugs such as β blockers, angiotensin converting enzyme inhibitors, antiarrhythmics, and sedatives—should be corrected if possible. Metabolic acidosis secondary to tissue hypoxia should be managed by treating the cause. Bicarbonate should be given only for severe acidosis that fails to respond to apparently adequate resuscitation.

If signs of shock persist despite volume replacement, and perfusion of vital organs is jeopardised, inotropic or other vasoactive agents may be given to improve cardiac output and blood pressure. The effects of a particular drug in an individual patient are unpredictable and the response must be closely monitored. In many cases this requires pulmonary artery catheterisation. Some patients are given inotropes or vasopressors to restore cardiac output and blood pressure, while in others inodilators are used to redistribute blood flow—for example, dopexamine to improve splanchnic perfusion.

What level of cardiac output is appropriate?

Although resuscitation has conventionally aimed at achieving normal haemodynamic values, survival of many critically ill patients is associated with raised values for cardiac output, oxygen delivery, and oxygen consumption.

Raising these variables to supranormal values is associated with improved outcome in victims of major trauma and high risk surgical patients. The benefit may be mainly due to optimal expansion of the circulating volume with consequent improvements in oxygen delivery and regional flow. The strategy has no benefit when started after admission to intensive care.

Low output states

Cardiogenic shock

Such patients have extremely low cardiac output, often with high ventricular filling pressures and increased systemic vascular resistance. Dobutamine can be given to improve cardiac

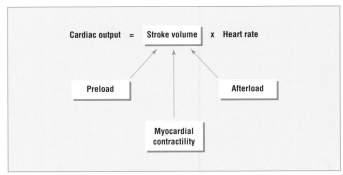

Determinants of cardiac output

Choice of fluid for volume replacement

- *Blood*—Clearly indicated in haemorrhagic shock and to maintain the haemoglobin concentration at an acceptable level (conventionally > 100 g/l or packed cell volume > 30%) in shock due to other causes
- *Crystalloids*—Cheap, convenient to use, and free of side effects but rapidly distributed across the intravascular and interstitial spaces; volumes 2-4 times that of colloid are required to achieve an equivalent haemodynamic response Moreover, volume expansion is transient, fluid accumulates in the interstitial spaces, and pulmonary oedema may result
- *Colloids* (starches, gelatins) produce a greater and more sustained increase in plasma volume with associated improvements in cardiovascular function and oxygen transport
- *Albumin* should be used only in special circumstances—for example, burns and children with septic shock

Receptor actions of sympathomimetic and dopaminergic drugs

	β₁	β₂	α₁	α₂	DA₁	DA₂
Adrenaline						
Low dose	+	+	+	±	NA	NA
Moderate dose	+ +	+	+ +	+	NA	NA
High dose	+ + (+)	+ + (+)	+ + + +	+ + +	NA	NA
Noradrenaline	+ +	0	+ + +	+ + +	NA	NA
Isoprenaline	+ + +	+ + +	0	0	NA	NA
Dopamine						
Low dose	±	0	±	+	+ +	+
Moderate dose	+ +	+	+ +	+	+ + (+)	+
High dose	+ + +	+ +	+ + +	+	+ + (+)	+
Dopexamine	+	+ + +	0	0	+ +	+
Dobutamine	+ +	+	±	?	0	0

NA = not applicable

> It is important to know the cardiovascular effects of available drugs and accurately assess haemodynamic disturbance before deciding on treatment

> Drugs with predominantly vasoconstrictor properties such as noradrenaline and, to a lesser extent, dopamine should be avoided in patients with cardiac failure

performance and reduce peripheral resistance; the heart rate usually increases and may contribute to the increase in cardiac output. The reduction in afterload and improved myocardial performance lowers ventricular filling pressures. Inodilators such as dopexamine, enoximone, and milrinone are alternatives.

Patients with cardiogenic shock or cardiac failure with pulmonary oedema may benefit from infusion of a vasodilator—eg, glyceryl trinitrate, isosorbide dinitrate, or sodium nitroprusside. Vasodilatation reduces afterload, thus increasing stroke volume and decreasing myocardial requirements by reducing systolic wall tension. Heart size and diastolic ventricular wall tension are reduced, improving coronary blood flow.

Intra-aortic balloon counterpulsation increases coronary blood flow and reduces left ventricular afterload. Myocardial ischaemia may be reversed and performance improved. This technique can support patients with cardiogenic shock who have surgically correctable lesions or those with low output states after heart surgery. It is less successful when cardiogenic shock complicates myocardial infarction and there is no surgically correctable lesion. It may also be considered for global myocardial dysfunction complicating anaphylaxis or septic shock.

Obstructive shock

Inotropic support may be indicated to maintain tissue perfusion until definitive treatment (pericardiocentesis for tamponade, thrombolysis for pulmonary embolism) relieves the underlying problem. With pulmonary embolism, expansion of the circulating volume should be combined with an inotropic agent that will maintain systemic blood pressure and thereby preserve right ventricular perfusion when right ventricular pressures are raised—eg, adrenaline or noradrenaline. In cardiac tamponade, vasodilatation and the associated fall in ventricular filling pressures could cause a large fall in cardiac output and blood pressure; these patients may also require vasoconstrictor drugs.

High output states

The dominant haemodynamic feature of distributive shock is peripheral vascular failure. In severe cases the vasodilatation is resistant to vasoconstrictors. Oxygen extraction and use is impaired. Provided that hypovolaemia has been corrected, cardiac output is usually high. Nevertheless, some myocardial depression is common in septic shock. Perfusion pressure can be restored by a vasoconstrictor such as noradrenaline, which may limit the degree of vasodilatation without compromising cardiac output. If required, dobutamine can be added to achieve an adequate cardiac output.

Adrenaline is cheap and effective but may cause lactic acidosis and aggravate splanchnic ischaemia. In less severe cases dopamine may be sufficient, although higher doses may be associated with worsening gut mucosal acidosis. Although dopexamine can increase heart rate and cardiac output in septic shock, systemic vascular resistance is further reduced and blood pressure falls. The value of inhibiting nitric oxide synthesis in septic shock, for example, with N^G-monomethyl-L-arginine (L-NMMA), is currently uncertain.

High risk surgical patients

Such patients benefit from intensive perioperative circulatory support, in particular maintenance of an adequate circulating volume, and postoperative care in intensive care. Morbidity and mortality have been reduced by preoperative admission to intensive care for optimisation of cardiovascular function. In such cases volume replacement and administration of inotropes or vasopressors should be guided by pulmonary artery catheterisation or an oesophageal Doppler probe.

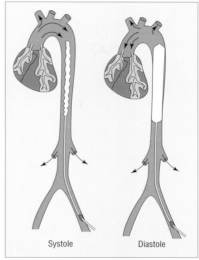

Intra-aortic balloon counterpulsation. A catheter with an inflatable balloon is inserted through a femoral artery into the descending thoracic aorta. The balloon is inflated early in diastole and deflated rapidly at the onset of systole

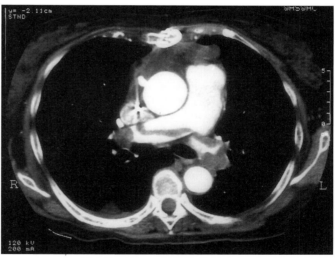

Computed tomogram of massive pulmonary emboli

Key points

- Treatment must be instituted early, before patients have developed irreversible peripheral vascular failure and defects in oxygen extraction or use
- Adequate volume replacement is essential in all cases
- Mean arterial pressure should be maintained at adequate levels, with reference to premorbid values
- Circulatory support should aim to achieve normal haemodynamics and restore tissue perfusion, while avoiding complications such as tachyarrhythmias, myocardial ischaemia, and exacerbation of microcirculatory abnormalities
- In patients with continued evidence of impaired tissue oxygenation moderate doses of inotropes may be given to further increase oxygen delivery. Aggressive use of inotropes to achieve supranormal values is no longer recommended

6   Renal support

Alasdair Short, Allan Cumming

Oliguria and renal dysfunction are common in critically ill patients. In most cases the kidney is an innocent bystander affected secondarily by the primary disease process. As patients with acute renal failure usually have multiple organ dysfunction and often require respiratory or circulatory support, they are increasingly referred to intensive care units rather than to specialist renal units. Nevertheless, close liaison with nephrologists is advisable, particularly when primary renal disease is suspected. It is rare for patients to develop acute renal failure after admission to intensive care unless a new problem has occurred or the primary process has not been controlled.

> **Renal failure is not an acceptable cause of death unless a conscious decision has been made not to treat it in the face of another non-recoverable disease**

Physiology

Urine is produced by glomerular filtration, which depends on the maintenance of a relatively high perfusion pressure within the glomerular capillary and an adequate renal blood flow.

Glomerular blood flow is autoregulated by the pre-glomerular arteriole until the mean arterial pressure falls to 80 mm Hg. Below this pressure the flow decreases. The autoregulation is achieved by arteriolar dilatation (partly mediated by prostaglandins and partly myogenic) as pressure falls and by vasoconstriction as pressure rises. If perfusion pressure continues to fall glomerular filtration pressure is further maintained by constriction of post-glomerular arterioles, which is mediated by angiotensin II.

The proximal tubules reabsorb the bulk of the filtered solute required to maintain fluid and electrolyte balance, but elimination of potassium, water, and non-volatile hydrogen ions is regulated in the distal tubules. As renal perfusion and glomerular filtration diminish, reabsorption of water and sodium by the proximal tubules rises from approximately 60% of that filtered to over 90% so that minimal fluid reaches the distal tubule. This explains why hypotensive or hypovolaemic patients cannot excrete potassium, hydrogen ions, and water. Similar defects in excretion of potassium and hydrogen ions occur in patients with distal tubular damage caused by drugs or obstructive uropathy.

The energy required for tubular function comes from aerobic metabolism within the mitochondria of the tubular cells. Tubular cells deep within the medulla operate at the limit of oxidative metabolism and are particularly sensitive to the effects of ischaemia and hypoxia. Blood flow to the medulla is threatened as renal perfusion falls and is maintained by the action of prostaglandins produced by the medullary interstitial cells. The cells of the thick ascending limb of the loop of Henlé are the most metabolically active in the deep medulla and thus the most vulnerable.

Role of kidneys in maintaining the internal environment

- Elimination of water soluble waste products of metabolism other than carbon dioxide
- Control of fluid and electrolyte homeostasis
- Elimination of water soluble drugs
- Endocrine function (erythropoietin, vitamin D, renin)

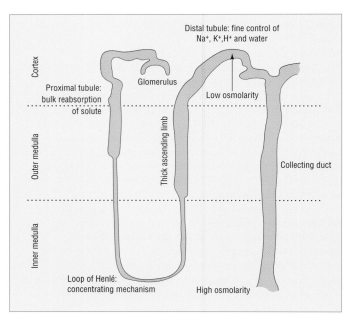

Diagram of nephron and position within kidney

Acute renal failure

Acute renal failure is defined as a sudden, normally reversible impairment of the kidneys' ability to excrete the body's nitrogenous waste products of metabolism. Acute renal failure is usually accompanied by oliguria. However, a daily urine volume above 500 ml does not necessarily imply normal renal function in critically ill patients. The plasma urea concentration rises with the breakdown of soft tissue or blood (which may be within the gut) or a high protein intake. Uraemia is a less reliable indicator of underlying renal function than creatinine

Criteria for diagnosis of acute renal failure

- Fall in urine volume to less than 500 ml per day
- Rising plasma urea and creatinine concentrations
- Rising plasma potassium and phosphate plus falling calcium and venous bicarbonate

concentration. The rate of production of creatinine is related to lean body mass, except in rhabdomyolysis. The concentration of creatinine in the blood reaches the upper limit of normal after 50% of function is lost and then doubles for each further 50% reduction in renal function.

Urine dipstick testing can detect haematuria and proteinuria, which may signify primary renal disease or other systemic disease. If primary glomerular disease is suspected a urine sample should be sent for microscopy. Although there are now direct tests for myoglobinuria, microscopy can help diagnose rhabdomyolysis and haemolysis. The stick test is strongly positive for haem pigment but no red cells are visible' on microscopy.

Simultaneous measurement of urinary and plasma urea, creatinine, and sodium concentrations and osmolality may help differentiate physiological oliguria of renal hypoperfusion from acute renal failure. Concurrent drug treatment—for example, diuretics or dopamine—will make values difficult to interpret. However, the findings will not generally alter management greatly. Patients with absolute anuria must be assumed to have lower urinary tract obstruction until proved otherwise. Always remember to check for a blocked catheter.

Established acute renal failure is confirmed by the lack of response to correction of any cardiorespiratory deficit, urinary tract obstruction, or septic process and rising concentrations of urea and creatinine. In critically ill patients it commonly results from a number of combined insults: hypovolaemia (absolute or relative), impaired renal perfusion (low perfusion pressure, low cardiac output), sepsis, drugs (including radiocontrast agents), hepatic dysfunction, obstruction of the collecting system (partial or complete), vascular occlusion (large or small vessel), or primary renal disease.

Standard guidelines exist for intensive care of patients with established or impending renal dysfunction. A window of opportunity exists between the onset of the insult(s) and the onset of established acute renal failure. Rapid identification and correction of these insults is essential and further potential insults must be avoided.

Correct circulation
Once hypoxaemia has been corrected (by using controlled ventilation if necessary) meticulous attention must be paid to cardiovascular function. Adequate intravascular volume, cardiac output, and perfusion pressure must be ensured before patients are given any diuretic or other drug purported to generate production of urine.

Correct metabolic acidosis
Severe metabolic acidosis secondary to renal tubular dysfunction can be corrected over 24-36 hours with isotonic sodium bicarbonate provided that the patient does not have a salt overload. Acidosis related to tissue hypoxia should be treated by addressing the underlying cause.

Exclude and relieve any urinary tract obstruction
Any obstruction at the bladder neck or urethra is relatively easily corrected by urethral or suprapubic catheterisation. Obstructions of the upper collecting system can be relieved at the bedside by percutaneous nephrostomy under ultrasonography.

Nephrotoxic drugs
Directly nephrotoxic drugs such as aminoglycosides should be avoided when possible. If they are given, blood concentrations should be measured regularly. Many drugs indirectly affect renal function by their effects on the circulation, and their

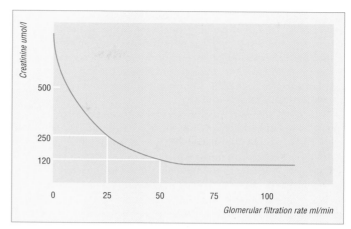

Relation of serum creatinine concentration to glomerular filtration rate

Investigations that may help to differentiate renal hypoperfusion from acute renal failure in oliguric patients

Measurement	Renal hypoperfusion	Acute renal failure
Fractional excretion of sodium (%)	< 1	> 4
Urinary sodium (mmol/l)	< 20	> 40
Urine:plasma urea ratio	> 20	< 10
Urine:plasma creatinine ratio	> 40	< 10
Urine:plasma osmolality ratio	> 2	< 1.2

Guidelines for immediate management of patients with oliguria or anuria

- Assess and correct any respiratory or circulatory impairment
- Manage any life threatening consequences of renal dysfunction (hyperkalaemia, salt and water overload, severe uraemia, extreme acidosis)
- Exclude obstruction of the urinary tract
- Establish underlying cause(s) and institute prompt remedial action
- Get a drug history and alter prescriptions appropriately
- Get help from senior appropriately trained specialists

The cause of acidosis will determine the treatment

- Tissue hypoxia/lactic acidosis—optimise circulation and oxygenation
- Salt and water depletion—normal saline
- Established renal failure (acute or chronic)—sodium bicarbonate, ?dialysis
- Poisoning (methanol, ethylene glycol, salicylate)—sodium bicarbonate, ?dialysis
- Liver failure—sodium bicarbonate, ?haemofiltration
- Diabetes mellitus—insulin, saline

concentration may build up as renal function deteriorates. In critically ill patients, especially those with sepsis, α and β adrenergic blocking drugs, angiotensin converting enzyme inhibitors, other vasodilators, and diuretics will potentiate any systemic circulatory disturbance and impair the intrarenal mechanisms that normally maintain glomerular filtration and medullary blood flow.

Non-steroidal anti-inflammatory drugs can produce an allergic interstitial nephritis, but more commonly in patients with a septic, systemic inflammatory, or hypovolaemic insult they impair the compensatory mechanisms that maintain glomerular perfusion and medullary blood flow to the ascending limb of the loop of Henlé. A single dose may be sufficient to precipitate failure of a stressed kidney. These drugs are thus contraindicated in critically ill patients.

Other drugs
The pharmacokinetics of many other drugs in critically ill patients with renal failure have not been established. Care must be taken with all drug treatment.

Renal protection
No convincing evidence exists that any of the regimens advocated to protect against or reverse renal failure are superior to salt loading (that is, extracellular fluid volume expansion with saline) and providing optimal renal perfusion (pressure as well as flow).

Mannitol has been suggested for situations such as obstructive biliary disease and vascular surgery, but there is little evidence that it is better than salt loading in humans other than for producing diuresis. In rhabdomyolysis, mannitol combined with aggressive salt loading and alkalinisation of the urine has been shown to reduce the incidence of severe renal damage.

Low dose dopamine has not been shown to improve renal function (glomerular filtration rate not diuresis) in randomised trials. If it does not have a diuretic effect within 24 hours it should be stopped. The use of loop diuretics to reduce oxygen requirements in the distal tubule in the stressed kidney is theoretically attractive but unproved.

Renal replacement therapy
Renal replacement therapy should be started early for patients who present with an absolute indication. The concentration of plasma urea at which renal replacement therapy should be started depends on the patient's condition. A patient with single organ failure secondary to a nephrotoxin might not require renal replacement therapy until the urea concentration is well above 30 mmol/l, but a patient with severe intra-abdominal sepsis such as faecal peritonitis with established renal failure should be treated early as urea concentrations will rise rapidly.

Most critically ill patients in the United Kingdom are now treated by semicontinuous methods of haemofiltration with or without dialysis rather than by short term haemodialysis as used in chronic renal replacement therapy. Peritoneal dialysis is used increasingly rarely in intensive care. Semicontinuous methods of treatment cause less fluctuation in the patient's biochemistry, which seems to improve cardiovascular stability. However, it has been difficult to prove that patient outcome has been affected other than in the presence of cerebral oedema—for example, in liver failure. The problems of obtaining access for extracorporeal circuits have been considerably reduced by the use of multilumen percutaneous venous catheters.

Nutrition
Critically ill patients should not be starved or have their protein intake restricted in an attempt to avoid renal replacement

---

Drugs that induce renal damage

Damage	Class of drug
Decrease in renal perfusion	Diuretics, angiotensin converting enzyme inhibitors, β blockers, vasodilators
Impaired intrarenal haemodynamics	Non-steroidal anti-inflammatories, radiocontrast agents
Tubular toxicity	Aminoglycosides, amphotericin, cisplatin
Allergic interstitial nephritis	β lactams, non-steroidal anti-inflammatories

---

Drugs that may cause acute interstitial nephritis in intensive care

- Antibiotics
  β lactams
  Rifampicin
  Sulphonamides
  Vancomycin
- Diuretics
  Thiazides
  Frusemide (furosemide)
- Non-steroidal anti-inflammatory drugs
- Others
  Ranitidine
  Cimetidine
  Phenytoin

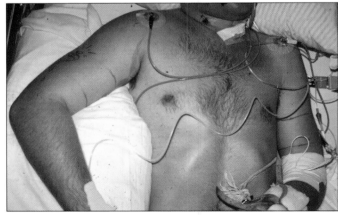

Rhabdomyolysis of shoulder and upper arm after prolonged compression secondary to overdose of tricyclic antidepressants. Note the pressure marks close to the axilla

---

Indications for renal replacement therapy

- Uncontrollable hyperkalaemia
- Severe salt and water overload unresponsive to diuretics
- Severe uraemia
- Acidaemia

therapy. It is better to accept the need for renal replacement therapy and allow appropriate nutrition. Specially formulated "renal" feeds have no advantage over standard feeding compounds in critically ill patients.

Recovery

The recovery phase is marked by an increase in urine volume as the nephrons recover and renal replacement therapy can be stopped. However, vigilance is still required as the kidney will have a reduced ability to conserve sodium, potassium, bicarbonate, and water. Modern management has made massive electrolyte and water losses uncommon. They may still occur after the relief of urinary tract obstruction because of the severe chronic distal tubular damage. Nephrotoxins and vasoactive drugs must be used with care, and non-steroidal anti-inflammatory drugs should be avoided. Renal function will usually return to within 90% of normal by 6 months after recovery from critical illness.

Patients with pre-existing chronic renal failure have a limited ability to conserve electrolytes and water which depends on their residual functioning renal mass. They cannot concentrate their urine to the normal level and may have an obligatory urine volume of up to 3 litres a day. As their intrarenal vascular compensatory mechanisms are continuously activated, they are more vulnerable to any insult. Careful attention to circulatory stability, electrolyte and water balance, and drug administration is essential.

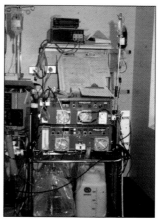

Semicontinuous haemofiltration

Key points

- Circulation must be corrected before any other specific intervention is started
- The cause of renal dysfunction must be determined and if possible treated
- Renal replacement therapy should be started and tailored according to the degree of biochemical derangement and the patient's underlying condition
- Primary renal disease is rare in critically ill patients but requires prompt referral to a nephrologist to avoid irreversible renal failure

7   Neurological support

Ian S Grant, Peter J D Andrews

The neurological conditions that require management in intensive care are diverse. Indications for admission range from maintaining the airway to control of seizures and intracranial pressure. Intensive care of a patient with a neurological disease requires a partnership between the referring specialist and intensive care doctors. Despite the diversity of the neurological diseases being managed some standard principles apply.

Acute brain injury and encephalopathy

Patients with acute brain injury, regardless of the cause, all raise similar intensive care problems. Some care, including ventilation, control of intracranial and cerebral perfusion pressure, and anticonvulsant treatment, may be similar, although patients will also require specific treatment of their condition. Patients should have their pupil size and responses assessed and conscious level measured by the Glasgow coma scale. These signs should be reassessed regularly thereafter.

Aims of intensive care management
The number and duration of secondary insults affect outcome. In particular, hypotension, decreased cerebral perfusion pressure, hypoxaemia, and hyperthermia are associated with a worse outcome. Intensive care management aims to avoid secondary insults and to optimise cerebral oxygenation by ensuring a normal arterial oxygen content and by maintaining cerebral perfusion pressure above 70 mm Hg. This figure may be modified depending on the jugular bulb oxygen saturation. Intracranial pressure should generally be below 25 mm Hg.

Intubated patients need sedation to avoid rises in intracranial pressure. Brain injured patients are prone to early nosocomial chest infection, due to impaired upper airway reflexes, and broad spectrum antibiotic prophylaxis may be advisable.

Sedation and paralysis
Sedation is required to depress coughing and spontaneous respiratory efforts in response to intubation and ventilation. Sedation depresses the cerebral metabolic rate and may improve the cerebral oxygen supply:demand ratio. A benzodiazepine (midazolam) is usually infused in combination with a short acting opioid such as alfentanil. Intravenous propofol can be used for depression of the cerebral metabolic rate, which coupled with cerebral vasoconstriction reduces intracranial pressure. However, it may also substantially reduce mean arterial pressure.

Patients with severe head injury generally require neuromuscular paralysis for the initial 12-24 hours in intensive care to prevent uncontrolled rises in intrathoracic and hence intracranial pressure. Thereafter, relaxants can be allowed to wear off. If patients remain well sedated without a rise in intracranial pressure they may be left unparalysed.

Specific monitoring techniques
The final common pathway in all acute brain injury is thought to be failure of oxygen delivery—that is, ischaemia. Monitors have been developed to detect critical falls in oxygen delivery.

Intracranial pressure monitoring—Most centres now use intraparenchymal monitors that are usually placed into the right (non-dominant) frontal region through a small burr hole. Although the intracranial pressure is important (normally

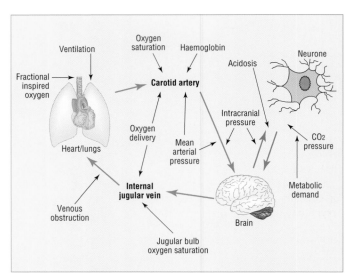

Interdependence of systemic and cerebral oxygen delivery variables

24

< 10 mm Hg, acceptable upper limit 25 mm Hg), the cerebral perfusion pressure is more important. It is calculated as mean arterial pressure minus intracranial pressure. Cerebral perfusion pressure is the principal determinant of cerebral blood flow.

Jugular bulb oxygen saturation monitoring—Bedside measurement of cerebral blood flow is difficult, but the jugular bulb oxygen saturation (Sjo_2) gives an indication of cerebral blood flow in relation to cerebral metabolic oxygen demand. The normal range is 50-75%. Low values indicate increased oxygen extraction, possibly due to low cerebral perfusion pressure or hyperventilation, while high values indicate cerebral hyperaemia. Monitoring jugular bulb oxygen saturation allows assessment of the effect of interventions on cerebral perfusion.

Transcranial Doppler ultrasound through a "window" in the temporal bone can be used to measure blood flow velocity in the basal cerebral arteries. The technique gives an indication of cerebral perfusion pressure and the presence of cerebral vessel narrowing if extracranial internal carotid velocities can be assessed (Lindegaard index).

Brain tissue oxygenation ($PBro_2$)—Regional estimates of oxygen pressure obtained by miniature Clark electrodes placed within cerebral tissue have been shown to correlate with outcome.

Processed electroencephalographic monitoring—Full electroencephalographic monitoring is generally too complex for routine use in intensive care. Various methods of electroencephalographic processing exist to allow assessment of cerebral electrical activity, detection of seizures, and titration of barbiturates or other anaesthetic treatment. Excessive anaesthetic infusion results in an isoelectric "flat" trace.

Cerebral protection

Considerable effort and funding have gone towards developing a neuroprotective drug to reduce mortality after brain trauma and improve functional recovery. There have been many failed or inconclusive studies, and the future of pharmacological neuroprotection after traumatic brain injury is in doubt. There is no evidence to support the use of corticosteroids after traumatic brain injury or routine use of profound hyperventilation ($Paco_2 < 3.3$ kPa). At best, these treatments do no good, and they may adversely affect outcome.

Clinicians managing patients with a head injury are therefore left with detection and prevention of secondary insults to the brain, including management of medical complications of brain injury and non-pharmaceutical interventions that might improve the brain's response to trauma. Of the potential interventions, moderate hypothermia is the most promising.

Subarachnoid haemorrhage

The outcome from severe subarachnoid haemorrhage has been poor. An aggressive approach based on intensive care and early surgical or endovascular intervention may improve outcome.

In general, principles of management are similar to those in traumatic brain injury, although specific management may be required for neurogenic pulmonary oedema—for example, pulmonary artery catheterisation and inotrope therapy. Patients with acute hydrocephalus require early drainage. Cerebral angiography and surgical clipping or coil embolisation should be considered early after cardiovascular control and adequate oxygenation have been achieved.

Delayed neurological deficit

Systemic therapy—All patients with subarachnoid haemorrhage should receive the calcium channel blocker nimodipine; however, caution is needed in haemodynamically

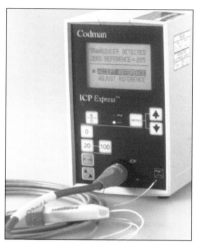

Solid state intraparenchymal intracranial pressure monitor

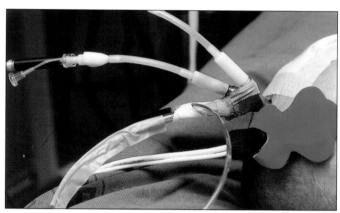

Brain tissue oxygenation, temperature, and pressure are measured by three probes through one burr hole. A near infrared spectroscopy optode is placed on the frontal region of the scalp and insulated from incident light

All neurological intensive care units require 24 hour access to computed tomography

Indications for intensive care for patients with head injury

- Not obeying commands after resuscitation and before intubation and ventilation or neurosurgical intervention
- Associated chest injury or multiple injuries that prevent continued assessment of head injury
- Unable to maintain airway or gas exchange
- Spontaneous hyperventilation ($Paco_2 < 3.5$ kPa)
- Repeated seizures

Indications for intensive care in subarachnoid haemorrhage

- Poor grade aneurysmal subarachnoid haemorrhage
- Rapidly decreasing Glasgow coma score or focal neurological deficit
- Complications, including cardiorespiratory dysfunction and particularly neurogenic pulmonary oedema (characterised by acute, severe, but reversible left ventricular dysfunction with associated pulmonary oedema)
- Delayed neurological deficit

unstable patients. In addition, patients should be actively hydrated; a combination of hypervolaemia, hypertension (using noradrenaline or dopamine), and haemodilution may reverse delayed neurological deficit. Early definitive treatment of the aneurysm—that is, before 96 hours—allows induction of hypertension without the risk of rebleeding.

Local therapy—Re-angiography and treatment for local arterial narrowing may be considered. Papaverine, nitroprusside, angioplasty, and thrombolysis have all been successful.

Duration of intensive care
In general, sedation and ventilation are maintained for at least 48 hours after brain injury, by which time evidence of brain swelling will be present. Ventilation should be continued until interventions to control intracranial pressure have not been needed for 24 hours. This may take 10-14 days of intensive care.

Acute ischaemic stroke
Increasing public awareness and early computed tomography will allow more aggressive management including thrombolysis and, in selected cases, intensive care.

Spinal cord injury

Physiological regulation of blood flow in the spinal cord is the same as for cerebral blood flow. Thus, most of the principles for managing traumatic brain injury apply to spinal cord injury.

Initial injury is associated with haemodynamic instability and cardiac arrhythmias, reportedly because of sympathetic stimulation. This is followed by the sudden onset of hypotension; loss of vasomotor tone is compounded in lesions above T2-T5, when sympathetic outflow to the heart is lost and parasympathetic tone is unopposed. The result is cardiac dysfunction, hypotension, and bradycardia. Spinal shock can last from weeks to months and is best managed in experienced intensive care units. Once reflex activity has returned below the level of the lesion autonomic dysreflexia can occur. Improvements in initial resuscitation, with early administration of high dose methylprednisolone, have improved functional recovery.

Peripheral neuropathies and neuromuscular and muscle disorders

The main conditions for which patients require intensive care are Guillain Barré syndrome and myasthenia gravis. Patients with other motor neuropathies, polymyositis, and muscular dystrophies may also require admission. Most patients are referred to intensive care with acute respiratory failure.

Patients at risk of developing respiratory failure should have pulse and respiratory rate measured hourly together with regular observation of chest movements and air entry and assessment of vital capacity. Pulse oximetry is useful when supplemental oxygen therapy is unnecessary, but a fall in oxygen saturation is a late sign in patients receiving oxygen. Patients with a vital capacity < 1.5 litre need their arterial blood gases checked. A vital capacity < 1 litre implies an inadequate cough.

Endotracheal intubation is indicated when impaired airway control (either as a result of bulbar dysfunction or inadequate cough) leads to an increased risk of aspiration. Most patients requiring intubation will need ventilation, as will patients with hypoxaemia or hypercapnia.

Mortality from Guillain Barré syndrome in intensive care is 3-8%, mainly because of avoidable complications. Problems include autonomic neuropathy, sepsis, constipation, deep

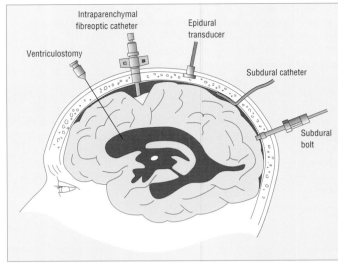

Sites of measurement of intracranial pressure

Perfusion pressure (mean arterial pressure minus cerebrospinal fluid pressure) is the main determinant of blood flow in the spinal cord

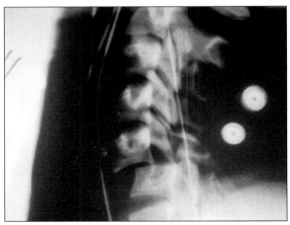

Lateral radiograph of unstable neck injury

Causes of acute respiratory failure in peripheral neurological disease

- Global respiratory muscle failure leading to inadequate alveolar ventilation and hypercapnia
- Fall in vital capacity due to muscle weakness resulting in failure to cough and clear secretions. This may cause acute respiratory failure due to bronchial obstruction and lobar or segmental collapse
- Bulbar dysfunction leading to failure of swallowing and coughing with consequent aspiration

---

Useful drugs for intubated patients with peripheral neuromuscular problems

Problem	Suggested treatment
Anxiolysis	Nasogastric diazepam
Neuropathic pain	Amitriptyline or carbamazepine
Musculoskeletal pain	Non-steroidal anti-inflammatory drugs
Initial artificial airway discomfort	Morphine

venous thrombosis, and depression. Scrupulous infection surveillance and careful electrocardiographic and haemodynamic monitoring are therefore essential.

Critical illness polyneuropathy

Critical illness polyneuropathy is a potential complication in patients with sepsis and multiple organ failure. It can result in areflexia, gross muscle wasting, and failure to wean from the ventilator. It therefore prolongs the period of intensive care.

Seizures

Prolonged or recurrent tonic-clonic seizures persisting for over 30 minutes (status epilepticus) constitute a medical emergency and require rapid treatment. Failure to control the seizures will result in massive catecholamine release, hypoxaemia, increased cerebral metabolism, hyperpyrexia, and hyperglycaemia.

Most patients respond to standard treatment—that is, oxygen, airway maintenance, and intravenous diazepam 5 mg, repeated if required. The cause of the seizures should be pursued and treated when appropriate—for example, glucose, calcium, or high dose vitamin B. If the seizures are not controlled with diazepam, or the patient develops hypoxaemia or loss of airway integrity, intravenous anaesthesia, endotracheal intubation, and ventilation are required. Thiopentone is the standard anaesthetic and is titrated until a burst suppression pattern is seen in processed electroencephalograms. Propofol is an alternative. It has the advantage that consciousness rapidly returns after it is stopped because it is quickly metabolised. Patients not already receiving therapeutic doses of phenytoin or other anticonvulsants should be loaded and the propofol or thiopentone dose maintained until therapeutic levels are achieved.

Outcome

Traumatic coma

Doctors and families of patients in coma face a difficult decision when considering whether life extending care will achieve a desirable outcome. Functional recovery can be assessed using the five point Glasgow outcome scale or the more detailed SF-36 health survey questionnaire. Sophisticated measures of functional recovery have also been developed.

Non-traumatic coma

Development of out of hospital resuscitation and improved training of paramedical staff have resulted in an increase in the number of patients in coma after cardiac arrest. Reliable prognosis can be achieved by assessing five variables in the first 3 days after insult. Abnormal brain stem reflexes and absent motor response best predict functional outcome.

After intensive care

Most patients require extra nursing, medical, and paramedical support after intensive care. A diminished level of consciousness or irritability in patients who have had acute brain injury may make nursing difficult. A tracheostomy is often required for aspiration of tracheobronchial secretions, while continuous positive airways pressure is needed to maintain basal lung expansion in the absence of spontaneous large tidal volume sighs. In patients with impaired consciousness and bulbar dysfunction, a percutaneous endoscopically guided gastrostomy may help feeding. All patients require a huge input from physiotherapists, speech therapists, occupational therapists, and nurses for full rehabilitation.

Effects of persistent seizures

- Cerebral and systemic hypoxia
- Lactic acidosis
- Neurogenic pulmonary oedema
- Rhabdomyolysis
- Hyperkalaemia
- Renal failure
- Hepatic necrosis
- Disseminated intravascular coagulation

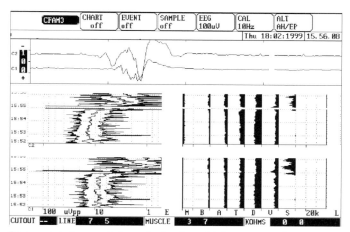

Processed electroencephalograph of patient with burst suppression pattern

---

Main determinants of outcome of traumatic coma

- Age
- Glasgow coma score after resuscitation
- Computed tomographic diagnosis
- Brain stem responses (pupil reaction)
- Presence of hypotension and hypoxia

Variables for assessing outcome of non-traumatic coma

- Abnormal brain stem responses
- Absent withdrawal response to pain
- Absent verbal response
- Plasma creatinine concentration >132.6 µmol/l
- Age ≥70 years
  Patients with 4-5 of these risk factors at 72 hours have a 97% mortality at 2 months

---

8 Other supportive care

Sheila Adam, Sally Forrest

As well as specific organ support techniques such as mechanical ventilation and renal replacement therapy, patients in intensive care require other interventions to maintain organ function and prevent further damage. These include nutritional support, preserving skin integrity, psychological support, and mobilisation. These interventions enable patients to recover their previous level of health, prevent intercurrent problems such as nosocomial infection and lung atelectasis, and support psychological and physical wellbeing.

Chest physiotherapy

Patients who are intubated or mechanically ventilated require chest physiotherapy to remove excess bronchial secretions, re-expand atelectatic areas, improve ventilation, decrease ventilation-perfusion mismatch, and mobilise the thoracic cage.

Bronchial secretions increase in intubated patients as the tracheal mucous membrane is irritated. These secretions may become tenacious as the patients' natural humidification has been bypassed. Expectoration may also be reduced by an ineffective cough, decreased ciliary action, and loss of sigh breaths.

Secretion tenacity can be reduced by adequate humidification and systemic hydration. Clearance of secretions is achieved by chest physiotherapy, suctioning, and occasionally bronchial lavage.

The primary aims of chest physiotherapy are to improve gas exchange and prevent atelectasis and consolidation, which occur as a result of mucus plugging or infection. Patients are assessed daily and will receive the following treatments as appropriate.

Positioning—For postural drainage or to improve ventilation-perfusion matching.

Manual hyperinflation—A 2 litre manual inflation bag is used to deliver up to 1.5 times the patient's tidal volume. An inspired breath is delivered at a slow rate and held for a short period before releasing rapidly. Normal saline can be instilled before the breath. This technique reinflates atelectatic areas of lung and loosens secretions by improving collateral ventilation . This improves arterial oxygenation and lung compliance.

Manual techniques—Shaking and vibrations applied to the chest wall may loosen secretions in the airways.

Suction—Secretions are removed by applying 25-30 kPa of negative pressure through a catheter passed down the endotracheal tube to the level of the carina.

Some of these techniques may then be done by nursing staff to maintain the condition of the chest.

Mobilisation

The musculoskeletal system is designed to keep moving; it takes only seven days of bed rest to reduce muscle bulk by up to 30%. Immobility and muscle wasting in intensive care patients must be attended to after an initial assesment. Immobility may be caused by administration of sedative and neuromuscular blocking agents, neurological deficit, and general debilitation and weakness. Patients with cardiorespiratory instability may need to be immobilised for long periods. The use of restricting support technology—for example, haemofiltration or intra-aortic balloon counterpulsation—may also limit movement.

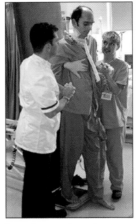

Intensive care is not just about organ support

Respiratory complications associated with tracheal intubation and mechanical ventilation

- Inability to clear secretions
- Trauma related to high inflation pressures, large tidal volumes, and shear stresses
- Microatelectasis and consolidation
- Alterations in ventilation-perfusion matching

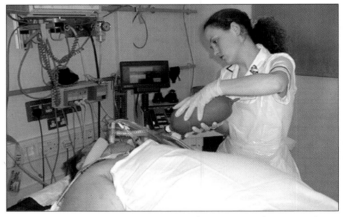

Manual hyperinflation improves lung compliance and arterial oxygenation

---

Disadvantages of immobility

Cardiovascular
- Venous stasis
- Increased risk of venous thrombosis and pulmonary embolism

Respiratory
- Decrease in functional residual capacity (when supine)
- Decreased lung compliance
- Retained secretions
- Atelectasis

Metabolic
- Increased excretion of nitrogen, calcium, potassium, magnesium, and phosphorus
- Osteoporosis
- Kidney stones

Musculoskeletal
- Decrease in muscle bulk
- Loss of bone density
- Decreased range of joint movement
- Pressure sores

Some patients develop critical illness polyneuropathy or myopathy after the acute phase of multiple organ dysfunction. This results in muscle wasting and often profound weakness. Affected patients exhibit flaccidity and a reduction or loss of deep tendon reflexes. Function is usually recovered, although it may take several months of rehabilitation.

Some patients may be able to undertake a partial active exercise regimen but most will require either active assisted or passive movements. These movements maintain full joint range, maintain full muscle length and extensibility, assist venous return, and maintain the sensation of normal movement.

Shoulders, hands, hips, and ankles are at particular risk of contractures. Resting splints for the hands and feet can be made or bought to maintain and protect these joints in a neutral position.

Early mobilisation out of bed is crucial even when the patient is intubated and ventilated. Hoists, tilt tables, and walking aids can be used to promote early physical rehabilitation.

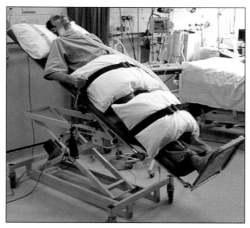
Tilt tables help early mobilisation

Pressure area problems

Patients not moved regularly will develop pressure sores on dependent areas. The most vulnerable areas are the tissues over bony prominences. Several factors associated with critical illness increase the likelihood of pressure sores.

Trauma and burns patients are at particular risk of pressure sores as are those with cardiovascular instability or diabetes. Preventive measures include regular turning and repositioning (usually every two to four hours). Special beds and mattresses should be used to relieve pressure over susceptible points and spread the pressure load in vulnerable patients. Regular inspection of the patient's skin integrity (especially high risk areas), early commencement of feeding, and prevention of contamination will all decrease the likelihood of problems.

Eye and mouth care

The mechanisms which normally protect mucosal and conjunctival surfaces exposed to the environment are lost to a greater or lesser degree in critically ill patients. Ventilated, sedated patients are often unable to blink or close their eyelids completely. There may be decreased tear production, a decreased resistance to infection, and a decrease in venous return with increased periorbital oedema due to rises in intrathoracic pressure associated with positive pressure ventilation.

The two commonest eye problems are dry eye and exposure keratopathy. The most effective measures are preventive. The corneal surface is kept moist by regularly applying artificial teardrops and hydrogel pads or tape to close the eyelids. Conjunctival oedema can be avoided by optimising ventilator settings, raising the patient's head, and ensuring that tapes securing the endotracheal tube are not too tight.

The incidence of buccal mucosal sores and infection is also increased because of a decreased or absent oral fluid intake, mucosal dehydration, decreased saliva production, the effects of drugs such as antibiotics, and the orotracheal tube hindering oral hygiene.

Mucosal care is also mainly preventive with frequent moisturising, teeth brushing, and removal of debris, saliva, and sputum. Oral candidiasis is common and requires early recognition and treatment with nystatin mouthwashes. Gingivitis should be treated with chlorhexidine mouthwashes.

Factors increasing likelihood of developing pressure sores in critically ill patients

- Inability to move
- Emaciation and muscle wasting
- Altered sensory function
- Depressed cardiac function
- Increased vasoconstriction
- Reduced peripheral perfusion

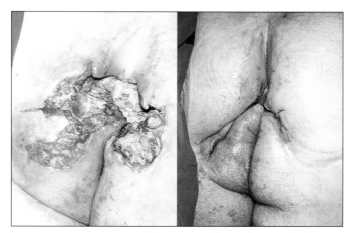
Severe pressure sores can usually be prevented by regular repositioning

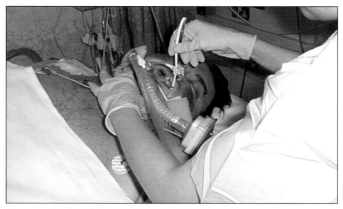
Good oral hygiene is important

Maintenance of nutritional intake

Most patients in intensive care are too sick to sustain an adequate oral diet. They therefore require enteral or parenteral nutrition, or a combination. The potential complications of parenteral nutrition mean that enteral feeding is attempted in most patients.

Unless there are specific reasons to the contrary, all patients likely to remain in intensive care for more than 48 hours should be started on enteral nutrition. Most patients can be enterally fed, sometimes with the use of prokinetic drugs.

A feeding protocol is a useful means of closing the gap between the volume of feed prescribed and that actually delivered to the patient. If patients cannot tolerate enteral nutrition, mixed feeding with minimal enteral feed plus parenteral supplementation or parenteral nutrition alone may be used.

Critically ill patients need about 0.7-1.0 g protein/kg/day, a minimum of 1 litre 10% fat emulsion weekly, and 83-146 kJ of non-protein energy/kg/day. Non-protein energy is usually given in a fat:carbohydrate ratio of 1:2.

Typical contents of enteral feeds (1.5-2.5 l /day)

Enteral feed (per 100 ml)	Energy (kJ)	Protein (g)	Sodium (mmol)	Potassium (mmol)
Standard	418	4	4	4
Energy dense*	627-836	5-8	4-5	4-5
Low sodium†	418	4	1.1	3.5
Low protein and minerals‡	836	2.8-4	1.5-4.3	2.8-3.8
High energy/low electrolytes§	836	7.0	3.4-4.3	2.7-3.8

*For high energy or protein requirements or fluid restriction.
†For serious hypernatraemia—for example, cardiac, renal, or liver failure.
‡For restricted fluid or protein and mineral intake—for example, hepatic encephalopathy.
§For patients on haemodialysis.

Typical composition of daily parenteral feed

Parenteral feed	Non-protein energy (MJ)	Nitrogen (g)	Sodium (mmol)	Potassium (mmol)	Calcium (mmol)	Magnesium (mmol)	Phosphate (mmol)
50 kg patient	6.7	9	80	60	5	7	28
70 kg patient	9.2	13.5	122.5	80	5	7	38

Absolute contraindications to enteral nutrition are gastrointestinal obstruction, prolonged paralytic ileus, and enterocutaneous fistulae. Relative contraindications include malabsorption and short bowel syndrome, inflammatory bowel disease, pancreatitis, and cholecystitis.

Increased infection risks

Patients in intensive care are five times more likely to develop a nosocomial infection than those on a general ward. Common sites of nosocomial infection are the lung, catheter puncture sites, urinary tract, and wounds. Three patterns of infection are seen:

Primary endogenous infection—the patient's own flora are the infecting organisms (for example, *Haemophilus influenzae*, *Streptococcus pneumoniae*, *Escherichia coli*).

Secondary (distant) endogenous infection—Caused by organisms from the throat or gastrointestinal tract (for example, *Acinetobacter* spp, *Serratia* spp, *Klebsiella*).

Exogenous infection—Direct transfer of organisms from the intensive care environment to the patient without passage through the throat or gut (such as *Staphylococcus* spp).

Mechanisms of infection include contamination of inspired air (through respiratory equipment), spread from neighbouring tissue, blood borne spread from a distant focus, and oropharyngeal-gastric colonisation followed by transfer to the trachea.

The most important preventive measure against the spread of infection is hand washing. As many as 40% of infections are transmitted on the hands of hospital staff.

Cross infection rates can be reduced by a vigorous infection control policy covering antibiotic use, timing and reasons for changing central venous catheters, isolation techniques, and use of disposable components (such as ventilator tubing and filters). Regular staff education and audit help to reinforce good practice.

Advantages and disadvantages of enteral and parenteral nutrition

	Advantages	Disadvantages
Enteral	More physiological	Diarrhoea in 24-40% of patients
	Cheaper	Difficulties in ensuring the amount prescribed is delivered
	Central venous access not required	Possible increased risk of nosocomial pneumonia
	Preserves gut mucosal integrity	Not tolerated by some patients
	May modify immune response to stress	
Parenteral	Does not require functioning gastrointestinal tract	Increased morbidity because of central venous access
	Easy to administer	Increased risk of infection
		Increased metabolic complications

Causes of increased risk of nosocomial infection

- Multiple vascular access sites
- Endotracheal tube bypassing mucous membranes and ciliary defences
- Sedation, mechanical ventilation, and immobility leading to pneumonia
- Indwelling urinary catheter
- Compromised immune function from critical illness, poor nutrition, underlying disease
- High numbers of critically ill patients in one area
- High use of antibiotics leading to bacterial resistance and fungal overgrowth

Preventing stress ulcers

The incidence of serious bleeding from stress ulcers in critically ill patients has fallen greatly in the past two decades. This is due to better overall patient management and greater attention to maintaining adequate organ perfusion and nutrition rather than to any specific treatment. A recent multicentre study suggested that ranitidine was superior to sucralfate with no increased risk of nosocomial pneumonia. Enteral feeding has been shown to be equally protective.

Psychological effects

Psychological disturbances associated with intensive care include sensory imbalance and disorientation. Patients may be confused, distracted, disoriented, restless, incoherent, agitated, or have hallucinations. There may be frank delirium, "intensive care unit psychosis," or acute anxiety disorders. There are numerous frightening or unpleasant stimuli such as pain, the presence of the endotracheal tube, disconnection from the ventilator, and sounding of ventilator, syringe pump, and monitor alarms. Patients may find the environment noisy, mechanistic, lacking in privacy, confined, and isolated. They may find it difficult to distinguish the passage of time, and dreams and hallucinations often have depersonalisation or torture themes.

Management is aimed at prevention of these problems. Staff should emphasise a clear difference between night and day by changing the ambient light. Natural light and windows at the patient's eye level are important design features. Clock faces should be large and easily visible, and patients should be surrounded by familiar objects, music, and family photos. Patients need repeated simple explanations about what is happening to them. Family participation in care and conversation is encouraged. Touch and human contact by both carers and family are also comforting and reassuring. As the patient's condition stabilises, lengthy periods of uninterrupted sleep are sought by clustering interventions; ensuring comfort by positioning, warmth, and analgesia; and reducing ambient noise and light. As the patient improves, control over the environment and independence should be encouraged.

If patients become disturbed, correctable causes such as catheter related infection should be sought. Patients can often be calmed verbally or with gentle yet firm touch. Sedatives or strong tranquillisers may be necessary to prevent the patient from self harm. Although agitation is obviously distressing, family and friends can be reassured that it is self limiting. It usually settles within a few days, and the patient often does not remember this acute confusional state.

Support of the family is also crucial and requires both skill and time. Relatives and friends are often traumatised by the patient's admission to intensive care and require comfort, information, and consideration in order to cope. Although they often feel frustrated and helpless during the acute phase of critical illness, they have a vital role in aiding recovery once the patient stabilises and regains awareness.

Up to two thirds of patients will have little or no recollection of their stay in intensive care. However, a small number will have clear memories and some will develop long term psychological disturbances. A post-traumatic stress disorder may occur, resulting in depression, sleep disturbances, and often vivid nightmares. Follow up clinics and psychological counselling for both patient and family are being introduced to help patients cope with the sequelae of their critical illness.

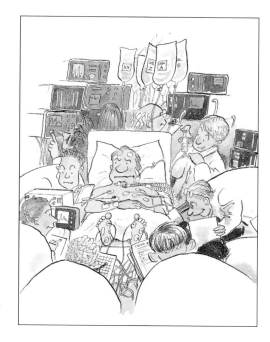

Causes of psychological disturbance
- Patients' illness—for example, head injury, sepsis, and hypotension
- Secondary complications such as nosocomial infection and electrolyte disorders
- Drugs and drug withdrawal— for example, sedatives, recreational drugs, alcohol
- Alien environment
- Loss of normal circadian rhythms and sleep patterns

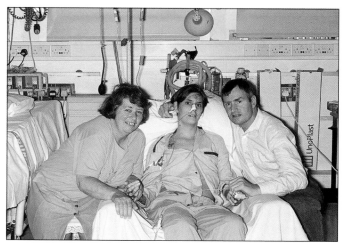
Family contact is reassuring

9 Outcome data and scoring systems

Kevin Gunning, Kathy Rowan

Intensive care has developed over the past 30 years with little rigorous scientific evidence about what is, or is not, clinically effective. Without these data, doctors delivering intensive care often have to decide which patients can benefit most. Scoring systems have been developed in response to an increasing emphasis on the evaluation and monitoring of health services. These systems enable comparative audit and evaluative research of intensive care.

Why are scoring systems needed?

Although rigorous experiments or large randomised controlled trials are the gold standard for evaluating existing or new interventions, these are not always possible in intensive care. For example, it is unethical to randomly allocate severely ill patients to receive intensive care or general ward care. The alternative is to use observational methods that study the outcome of care patients receive as part of their natural treatment. However, before inferences can be drawn about outcomes of treatment in such studies the characteristics of the patients admitted to intensive care have to be taken into account. This process is known as adjusting for case mix.

The death rate of patients admitted to intensive care units is much higher than that of other hospital patients. Data for 1995-8 on 22 057 patients admitted to 62 units in the case mix programme, the national comparative audit of patient outcome, showed an intensive care mortality of 20.6% and total hospital mortality of 30.9%. However, mortality across units varied more than threefold. Clearly, it is important to account for this variation.

Given the relatively high mortality among intensive care patients, death is a sensitive, appropriate, and meaningful measure of outcome. However, death can result from many factors other than ineffective care. Outcome depends not only on the input (equipment, staff) and the processes of care (type, skill, and timing of care) but also on the case mix of the patients. The patient population of an intensive care unit in a large tertiary centre may be very different from that of a unit based in a district general hospital. Patients are admitted to intensive care for a wide range of clinical indications; both the nature of the current crisis and any underlying disease must be considered. Intensive care units admitting greater proportions of high risk patients would be expected to have a higher mortality. For example, the risk of death would be higher for a 76 year old with chronic obstructive airways disease admitted with faecal peritonitis than for a 23 year old in diabetic coma.

Scoring systems

Various characteristics such as age have been recognised as important in increasing the risk of death before discharge from hospital after intensive care. It is essential to account for such patient characteristics before comparing outcome.

Scoring systems are aimed at quantifying case mix and using the resulting score to estimate outcome. Outcome has usually been measured as death before discharge from hospital after intensive care. In the mid-1970s William Knaus developed the APACHE (acute physiology and chronic health evaluation)

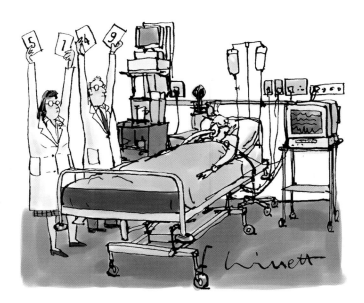

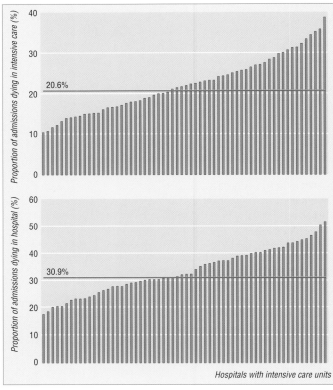

Distribution of intensive care unit and hospital mortality across hospitals

---

Factors increasing risk of death after intensive care

- Increasing age
- Greater severity of acute illness
- History of severe clinical conditions
- Emergency surgery immediately before admission
- Clinical condition necessitating admission

scoring system, which scored patients according to the acute severity of illness by weighting physiological derangement.

Initially, 34 physiological variables which were thought to have an effect on outcome were selected by a small panel of clinicians. These were then reduced to 12 more commonly measured variables for the APACHE II scoring system published in 1985. Up to four points are assigned to each physiological variable according to its most abnormal value during the first 24 hours in intensive care. Points are also assigned for age, history of severe clinical conditions, and surgical status. The total number of points gives a score ranging from 0-71, with an increasing score representing a greater severity of illness.

The reason for admission to intensive care has also been shown to affect outcome. As most intensive care units do not see a sufficient number of patients with the same condition, mathematical equations were developed to estimate probabilities of outcome derived from databases containing several thousand patients from many intensive care units. APACHE II allows the probability of death before discharge from hospital to be estimated. The probability of death for each patient admitted to intensive care can be summed to give the expected hospital death rate for the whole group. The expected hospital death rate can then be compared with the actual hospital death rate. This is often expressed as the standardised mortality ratio, the ratio of actual to expected deaths.

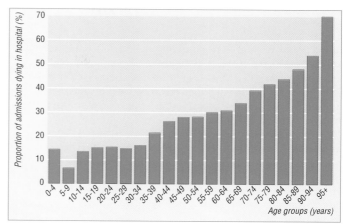

Relation of age to hospital mortality

Acute physiology and chronic health evaluation (APACHE II) scoring system

Physiology points	4	3	2	1	0	1	2	3	4
Rectal temperature (°C)	≥41.0	39.0-40.9		38.5-38.9	36.0-38.4	34.0-35.9	32.0-33.9	30.0-31.9	≤29.9
Mean blood pressure (mm Hg)	≥160	130-159	110-129		70-109		50-69		≤49
Heart rate (beats/min)	≥180	140-179	110-139		70-109		55-69	40-54	≤39
Respiratory rate (breaths/min)	≥50	35-49		25-34	12-24	10-11	6-9		≤5
Oxygenation (kPa)*:									
Fio$_2$ ≥50% A-aDo$_2$	66.5	46.6-66.4	26.6-46.4		<26.6				
Fio$_2$ <50% Pao$_2$					>9.3	8.1-9.3		7.3-8.0	<7.3
Arterial pH	≥7.70	7.60-7.59		7.50-7.59	7.33-7.49		7.25-7.32	7.15-7.24	<7.15
Serum sodium (mmol/l)	≥180	160-179	155-159	150-154	130-149		120-129	111-119	≤110
Serum potassium (mmol/l)	≥7.0	6.0-6.9		5.5-5.9	3.5-5.4	3.0-3.4	2.5-2.9		<2.5
Serum creatinine (μmol/l)	≥300	171-299		121-170	50-120		<50		
Packed cell volume (%)	≥60		50-59.9	46-49.9	30-45.9		20-29.9		<20
White blood cell count (×10⁹/l)	≥40		20-39.9	15-19.9	3-14.9		1-2.9		<1

*If fraction of inspired oxygen (Fio$_2$) is ≥50% the alveolar-arterial gradient (A—a) is assigned points. If fraction of inspired oxygen is <50% partial pressure of oxygen is assigned points.

Other points
Glasgow coma scale: Score is subtracted from 15 to obtain points.
Age <45=0 points, 45-54=2, 55-64=3, 65-75=5, ≥75=6.
Chronic health points (must be present before hospital admission): chronic liver disease with hypertension or previous hepatic failure, encephalopathy, or coma; chronic heart failure (New York Heart Association grade 4); chronic respiratory disease with severe exercise limitation, secondary polycythaemia, or pulmonary hypertension; dialysis dependent renal disease; immunosuppression—for example, radiation, chemotherapy, recent or long term high dose steroid therapy, leukaemia, AIDS. 5 points for emergency surgery or non-surgical patient, 2 points for elective surgical patient.

Proposed roles for scoring systems

Comparative audit
Comparisons of actual and expected outcomes for groups of patients can be used to compare different providers. It is assumed that a standardised mortality ratio greater than 1.0 may reflect poor care and, conversely, a ratio below 1.0 may reflect good care. The reasons for any unexpected results can

Proposed roles for scoring system

- Comparative audit
- Evaluative research
- Clinical management of patients

then be investigated locally. Review of deaths among patients estimated to be at lower risk of death may show that a particular group of patients or those discharged at a particular time of day have a poorer prognosis.

Evaluative research

When non-randomised or observational methods are used to evaluate interventions a valid means of adjusting for differences in case mix is needed. Accurate estimates of expected hospital death rates for groups of patients can be used in research studies to identify those components of intensive care structure and process that are linked to improved outcome.

Scoring systems have also been proposed to aid stratification in randomised controlled trials. Given the considerable heterogeneity of patients in intensive care stratification based on an accurate, objective estimate of the probability of death before hospital discharge should create a more homogeneous subset of patients and improve isolation of the effects of an intervention.

Clinical management of individual patients

Scores obtained from scoring systems have been proposed as a clinical shorthand—that is, a common, standard terminology to rapidly convey information about a patient. They have also been proposed for use in triage to classify patients according to severity of illness.

Although early scoring systems were designed only for comparing observed and expected outcomes, some of the second and third generation scoring systems are promoted as methods to guide clinical care and treatment. Such decisions might include when to withdraw treatment or when to discharge a patient. This proposal has generated considerable debate, even though scoring systems have been shown to be as good as clinicians in predicting survival. Some of the more recent methods have incorporated trend analysis to try to improve the ability to predict outcome for individual patients. However, current scoring systems provide only probabilities and do not accurately predict whether an individual will survive. They therefore should not be used alone to determine decisions about intensive care.

Types of scoring systems

Scoring systems in intensive care can be either specific or generic. Specific scoring systems are used for certain types of patient whereas generic systems can be used to assess all, or nearly all, types of patient. The scoring system may be either anatomical or physiological. Anatomical scoring systems assess the extent of injury whereas physiological systems assess the impact of injury on function. Scores from anatomical scoring systems, once assessed, are fixed whereas physiological scores may change as the physiological response to the injury or disease varies.

The first scoring systems were developed for trauma patients and were either specific anatomical methods (abbreviated injury score, 1969; burns score, 1971; injury severity score, 1974) or specific physiological methods (trauma index, 1971; Glasgow coma scale, 1974; trauma score, 1981; sepsis score, 1983).

The Glasgow coma scale is still in general use in intensive care. The scale avoids having to describe a patient's level of neurological function in words and the assumption that colleagues understand the same meaning from those words.

The later scoring systems developed for intensive care have been generic. Two main approaches have been used; one is aimed at measuring severity by treatment intensity and the second at measuring severity by patient characteristics and physiological measurements.

Estimation of probability of death in hospital by applying APACHE II for 71 year old man admitted to intensive care from the hospital's accident and emergency department with (a) abdominal aortic aneurysm and (b) asthma attack

Criteria	Value	Points
Primary reason for admission	(a) Abdominal aortic aneurysm	
	(b) Asthma attack	
Age	71 years	5
History	None	0
Physiology:		
Temperature	38.4°C	1
Mean blood pressure	112 mm Hg	2
Heart rate	136 beats/min	2
Respiratory rate	28 breaths/min	1
Oxygenation:		0
Fraction of inspired oxygen	0.4	
Partial pressure of oxygen	21.2 kPa	
Partial pressure of carbon dioxide	4.4 kPa	
pH	7.09	4
Serum sodium	150 mmol/l	1
Serum potassium	5.5 mmol/l	1
Serum creatinine	145 µmol/l	2
Packed cell volume	40%	0
White blood cell count	20×10^9/l	2
Glasgow coma score:		
Eyes	Opening spontaneous	
Motor	Obeys verbal command	1
Verbal	Disoriented and converses	
Total		**22**

(a) APACHE II probability of hospital death: Abdominal aortic aneurysm (0.731) + APACHE II score
$(22 \times 0.146 = 3.212) - 3.517 = 0.426$
$$\frac{e^{0.426}}{1 + e^{0.426}} = 0.6049182 = 60.5\% \text{ probability of hospital death}$$
(b) APACHE II probability of hospital death: Asthma attack in known asthmatic (-2.108) + APACHE II score
$(22 \times 0.146 = 3.212) - 3.517 = -2.413$
$$\frac{e^{-2.413}}{1 + e^{-2.413}} = 0.08211867 = 8.2\% \text{ probability of death}$$

Glasgow coma scale

Score	Eye opening	Motor	Verbal
6		Obeys commands	
5		Localises to pain	Oriented
4	Spontaneous	Flexes to pain	Confused
3	To speech	Abnormal flexor	Words only
2	To pain	Extends to pain	Sounds only
1	No response	No response	No response

The total score is the sum of the three variables.

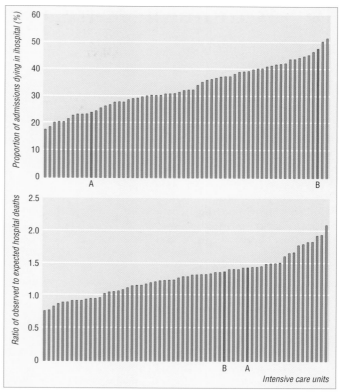

Measuring severity by treatment

The therapeutic intervention scoring system (TISS) published in 1974 was developed to quantify severity of illness among intensive care patients based on the type and amount of treatment received. The underlying philosophy was that the sicker the patient, the greater the number and complexity of treatments given. By quantifying this, a proxy measure of the severity of illness for a patient could be obtained. The system scored 76 common therapeutic activities and was last updated in 1983. A simplified version based on 28 therapeutic activities (TISS 28) has been published and a version for patients in high dependency units has been proposed.

Another approach is to assess the severity of organ dysfunction based on the type and amount of treatment received. These organ failure scoring systems are used to give a probability of hospital death which takes into account the severity of dysfunction in each organ system and the effect on prognosis of dysfunction in several organ systems.

Measuring severity by patient characteristics and physiological measurements

The first generic physiological scoring system developed to quantify severity of illness by patient characteristics was the APACHE method, described above. The original system was too complex and time consuming to collect routinely, so two derivations were developed—the simplified acute physiology score (SAPS) and the APACHE II system. These were both subsequently updated to APACHE III in 1991 and SAPS II in 1993. An alternative system is the mortality prediction model (MPM II).

Selecting a scoring system

The scoring system chosen depends on the proposed use. The main criteria for selection should be the accuracy (validity and reliability) of the score and the goodness of fit (calibration and discrimination) of the mathematical equation used to estimate outcome. Rigorous comparison of the accuracy and goodness of fit of most scoring systems has not been done in the United Kingdom. APACHE II has been tested and is the most widely used.

Outcome from intensive care

Although death before discharge from hospital is the usual measure of outcome, disability, functional health, and quality of life should not be ignored. A study published in 1994 showed that in the first year after discharge from intensive care the risk of patients dying was 3.4 times greater than that of a matched population; the excess risk did not disappear until the fourth year after discharge.

Quality of life after a critical illness has been measured by various methods. The results differ according to the method used and the types of patient studied. Age and pre-existing severe clinical conditions seem to greatly affect quality of life after intensive care. In one study, 62% of young trauma victims who survived intensive care reported significant severe social disability and modest to severe impairment at work 10 months after discharge. In contrast, another study of a mixed group of patients found that those with pre-existing severe clinical conditions showed some improvement in their quality of life 6 months after admission to intensive care. A systematic review of the literature is underway.

Hospital mortality and standardised mortality ratios across hospitals. The effect of case mix is important. Superficially, hospital death rates for patients admitted to intensive care unit B are higher than those for patients admitted to unit A. However, after adjustment for case mix the standardised mortality ratio is similar for both units

Criteria for selecting a scoring system

- Proposed use
- Validity of score
- Reliability of score
- Discrimination of scoring system
- Calibration of scoring system

35

10 Withdrawal of treatment

Bob Winter, Simon Cohen

All medical practice should be governed by basic ethical principles, and intensive care medicine is no exception. Indeed, because of the nature of intensive care ethical issues are addressed almost daily.

Ethical principles of medical care

- Autonomy
- Beneficence
- Non-maleficence
- Distributive justice

Why withdraw treatment?

Withdrawal of treatment is an issue in intensive care medicine because it is now possible to maintain life for long periods without any hope of recovery. Intensive care is usually a process of supporting organ systems, but it does not necessarily offer a cure. Prolonging the process of dying is not in the patient's best interests as it goes against the ethical principles of beneficence and non-maleficence. However, withdrawal of treatment does not equate with withdrawal of care. Care to ensure the comfort of a dying patient is as important as the preceding attempts to achieve cure.

It is often easier to withhold a treatment than to withdraw it once it has been instituted. Ethically, however, there is no difference between withdrawing a treatment that is felt to offer no benefit and withholding one that is not indicated. The common practice of offering a short period of aggressive intensive care in an attempt to gain improvement, followed by review, will inevitably mean that treatment is withdrawn for patients who have not improved and for whom death is felt to be inevitable.

About 70% of deaths in intensive care occur after withdrawal of treatment. This is not euthanasia. The cause of death remains the underlying disease process, and treatment is withdrawn as it has become futile. However, the timing of withdrawal, the treatments withdrawn, and the manner of withdrawal may vary considerably, not only from country to country but also between intensive care units in the same country.

Patient autonomy

Autonomy is another of the basic precepts of ethical practice, but there are problems with its implementation in the intensive care unit. Most critically ill patients are not competent to participate in discussion because of sedation or their illness. In some American states a designated chain of surrogacy exists. However, in the United Kingdom relatives do not have legal rights of decision making. Recent cases of conflict in the United States between healthcare providers and families have shown that the use of surrogates does not necessarily increase the chances of best care for the patient. Families may also find the concept of futile care difficult to accept. Furthermore, data on which prognoses are based are statistical and cannot necessarily be applied to an individual patient.

Another difficult issue occurs when a patient may survive but with a poor quality of life. The concept of "relative futility" is dangerous as it introduces an unknown and potentially highly variable factor—namely, a doctor's judgment on the patient's quality of life. Substitution of the word "reasonable" for "relative" has been argued to give doctors more latitude in deciding whether a treatment is ethically justifiable.

Dr A decides to continue but not increase the level of vasoactive drug support or inspired oxygen concentration given to a man with multiple organ failure who has been in intensive care for 16 days. Over the next 5 days the patient improves; noradrenaline is discontinued and ventilatory support reduced, and he begins to rouse. He then develops a probable catheter related sepsis and deteriorates. Should Dr A abide by his previous decision of non-escalation? If not, why did he make the decision in the first place? What would he do if treatment was restarted but a similar situation occurred a week later?

It would be appropriate (although it might be viewed as inconsistent) to review each requirement for treatment in the light of the patient's current condition

---

An 18 year old patient has chemotherapy and bone marrow transplantation for leukaemia. While waiting for marrow recovery she develops respiratory failure and needs mechanical ventilation with 100% oxygen. Shortly after she requires increasing doses of noradrenaline and progresses to anuric renal failure. The intensive care team suggest that treatment should be withdrawn as her chances of survival are remote, but the haematologists argue that her renal, respiratory, and cardiovascular failure are potentially reversible if the bone marrow is given time to recover. After discussion with the family it is agreed that treatment should be withdrawn on the grounds of futility

---

An Asian man is brought into hospital in a coma after a massive subarachnoid haemorrhage, which is confirmed by computed tomography. Despite full intensive care he becomes brain dead. The doctors approach the family about the possibility of organ donation, but they refuse on cultural grounds. They also refuse to permit withdrawal of support as their religion does not accept brain death. Should the family's wishes be respected or should support be withdrawn regardless?

It was decided to maintain full support until the patient died 5 days later

When to withdraw treatment

In general, treatment is withdrawn when death is felt to be inevitable despite continued treatment. This would typically be when dysfunction in three or more organ systems persists or worsens despite active treatment or in cases such as multiple organ failure in patients with failed bone marrow transplantation. These decisions remain difficult because of the paucity of data on different clinical scenarios.

Whatever the definition of futility used the carers must act as advocates for the patient. This requirement has, however, been criticised as paternalistic. Advance directives are uncommon in the United Kingdom. The advance refusal of treatment is legally binding provided certain conditions are met. The BMA has issued a statement supporting the use of living wills. A problem still exists unless they are precisely worded.

Caring for families

Regardless of whether families are involved in the decision making process, they are affected by the behaviour of the carers. Families who feel excluded from discussion, who have had the burden of decision making placed on them, or in cases where there was delay or excess haste in enacting decisions express negative feelings towards the process of withdrawing treatment. Communication with the family is a vital part of the general care of intensive care patients. Relatives must be kept fully informed about the patient's condition, in particular regarding issues of limiting and withdrawing treatment. Although decisions rest with the medical staff, it is unwise to limit or withdraw treatment without the agreement of the relatives.

Process of withdrawal

Approaches to the withdrawal of treatment vary with the attitudes of the intensive care doctors. Some doctors are prepared only to withhold treatment rather than to withdraw it despite the lack of ethical distinction. This approach can create difficulties once the threshold for the withheld treatment is reached.

Once a decision has been made to withdraw treatment and agreement has been obtained from the family and admitting team, inotropes and vasopressors are discontinued, sedation may be increased, and the inspired oxygen concentration reduced to room air. Other supportive treatments such as renal replacement therapy are also removed. Death usually follows shortly afterwards. Only rarely is ventilation discontinued.

In general, it is better for the family if the patient is not moved from intensive care once the decision is made. It is unfair to expose the family to unfamiliar staff at this distressing time, especially if they have built up a rapport with nursing and medical staff. Most units have rooms where the family can be with the patient.

Problems

Problems arising from decisions to withdraw treatment can be divided into four types.

The referring team request continued futile therapy
This can usually be resolved by explaining the rationale and offering a second opinion from another intensive care consultant. If conflict still remains, treatment cannot be withdrawn. The family should not be informed of a decision to withdraw that is then rescinded because of interteam conflicts. It will reduce their faith in subsequent decisions and undermine confidence in the predicted outcome.

Living Will
Advance Directives

1 - Medical treatment in general

Three possible health conditions are described below.

For each condition, choose 'A' or 'B' by ticking the appropriate box, or leave both boxes blank if you have no preference. The choice between 'A' or 'B' is exactly the same in each case.

Treat each case separately. You do not have to make the same choice for each one.

I declare that my wishes concerning medical treatment are as follows.

Case 1 - Life-threatening condition

Here are my wishes if:
- I have a physical illness from which there is no likelihood of recovery; *and*
- the illness is so serious that my life is nearing its end.

A I want to be kept alive for as long as is reasonably possible using whatever forms of medical treatment are available. ☐

B I do not want to be kept alive by medical treatment. I want medical treatment to be limited to keeping me comfortable and free from pain. I refuse all other medical treatment. ☐

Case 2 - Permanent mental impairment

Here are my wishes if:
- my mental functions have become permanently impaired;
- the impairment is so severe that I do not understand what is happening to me;
- there is no likelihood of improvement; *and*
- my physical condition then becomes so bad that I would need medical treatment to keep me alive.

A I want to be kept alive for as long as is reasonably possible using whatever forms of medical treatment are available. ☐

B I do not want to be kept alive by medical treatment. I want medical treatment to be limited to keeping me comfortable and free from pain. I refuse all other medical treatment. ☐

Case 3 - Permanent unconsciousness

Here are my wishes if:
- I become permanently unconscious and there is no likelihood I will regain consciousness.

A I want to be kept alive for as long as is reasonably possible using whatever forms of medical treatment are available. ☐

B I do not want to be kept alive by medical treatment. I want medical treatment to be limited to keeping me comfortable and free from pain. I refuse all other medical treatment. ☐

Living wills enable people to have a say in their treatment when they are incapable of taking part in decision making

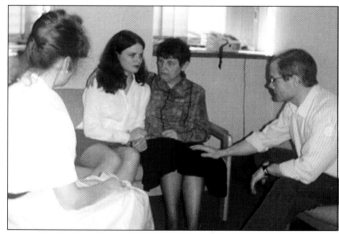

Talking to patients' relatives is best done in a quiet room of the unit

The patient's family requests continued futile therapy

Guilt usually plays a part in the family's request to continue treatment, although religious and cultural factors may also contribute. Agreement can usually be obtained by explaining the rationale again and offering a second opinion from within or outside the intensive care team. It is best not to withdraw treatment if there is conflict. However, the final decision rests with the intensive care team. This underlines the need for good communication.

The family requests inappropriate discontinuation of therapy

The rationale behind the therapy and the reasons why continuing treatment is thought appropriate should be explained. The duty of care is to the patient, not the family. Again, a second opinion can be offered.

The patient requests discontinuation of therapy.

Explain to the patient the rationale for the treatment and that, in the opinion of the intensive care team, a chance of recovery exists. It may be appropriate to offer a short term contract for treatment (for example, 48 hours then review). Ultimately, the competent patient has the right to refuse treatment even if that treatment is life saving.

The living will was provided by Terence Higgins Trust and King's College London.

A 65 year old man is admitted to intensive care after a laparotomy for faecal peritonitis secondary to a perforated diverticulum. He needs mechanical ventilation, haemofiltration, and noradrenaline. Two days later his children (the next of kin) request discontinuation of treatment as they feel that their father would not wish to be put through this suffering and had strongly expressed such views. However, he shows evidence of clinical improvement and his requirements for noradrenaline and oxygen are significantly reduced. The intensive care team therefore felt that treatment should not be withdrawn.

The man recovered and was discharged from hospital. It was later discovered that his family had apportioned his possessions while he was in intensive care

11 Transport of critically ill patients

Peter G M Wallace, Saxon A Ridley

Intensive care patients are moved within hospital—for example, to the imaging department—or between hospitals for upgraded treatment or because of bed shortages. We will concentrate on transport of adults between hospitals, but the principles are similar for transfers within hospitals.

Although the Intensive Care Society and the Association of Anaesthetists have recommended that retrieval teams are established in the United Kingdom, 90% of patients are accompanied by staff from the referring hospital. Over 10 000 intensive care patients are transferred annually in the United Kingdom, but most hospitals transfer fewer than 20 a year. Each hospital thus has little expertise and few people gain knowledge of transport medicine. Most patients are accompanied by on call anaesthetic trainees. Not only does this leave the base hospital with inadequate on call staff but accompanying doctors often have little experience.

Dangers of transport

Intensive care patients have deranged physiology and require invasive monitoring and organ support. Furthermore, they tend to become unstable on movement. Transport vehicles are not conducive to active intervention and no help is available. Staff and patients are vulnerable to vehicular accidents and may be exposed to temperature and pressure changes.

Audits in the United Kingdom suggest that up to 15% of patients are delivered to the receiving hospital with avoidable hypotension or hypoxia which adversely affects outcome. About 10% of patients have injuries that are undetected before transfer. However, with experienced staff, appropriate equipment, and careful preparation, patients can be moved between hospitals without deterioration. The "scoop and run" principle is not appropriate for moving critically ill patients.

Organisation

Each hospital should have a designated consultant responsible for transfers who ensures that guidelines are prepared for referral and safe transfer, equipment and staff are available, and standards are audited. Proper routines for referral between hospitals and good communication should ensure appropriate referral, coordination, and integration of services. An area or regional approach may allow retrieval teams to be established.

Transfer decisions

A decision to transfer should be made by consultants after full assessment and discussion between referring and receiving hospitals. Guidelines exist concerning timing of transfer for certain groups of patients—for example, those with head injury. For patients with multiple organ failure the balance of risk and benefit needs to be carefully discussed by senior staff.

The decision on whether and how to send or retrieve a patient will depend on the urgency of transfer, the availability and experience of staff, equipment, and any delay in mobilising a retrieval team. Local policies should be prepared to reflect referral patterns, available expertise, and clinical circumstances.

Principles of safe transfer
- Experienced staff
- Appropriate equipment and vehicle
- Full assessment and investigation
- Extensive monitoring
- Careful stabilisation of patient
- Reassessment
- Continuing care during transfer
- Direct handover
- Documentation and audit

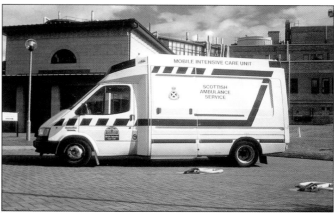

Specially equipped ambulances are best for transferring patients

---

Organisational structure

National and regional
Department of Health, purchasers, and specialist societies have responsibility for
- Guidelines
- Audit
- Bed bureau
- Funding
- Regional retrieval teams

Hospital or trust
Consultant with overall responsibility for transfers including
- Local guidelines, protocols, check lists
- Coordination with neighbouring hospitals
- Availability and maintenance of equipment
- Nominated consultant for 24 hour decisions
- Call out system for appropriate staff
- Indemnity and insurance cover
- Liaison with ambulance service concerning specification of vehicle and process of call out
- Communication systems between units and during transfer
- Education and training programmes
- Audit: critical incident, morbidity, and mortality
- Funding: negotiations with purchasers

Transfer vehicle

Vehicles should be designed to ensure good trolley access and fixing systems, lighting, and temperature control. Sufficient space for medical attendants, adequate gases and electricity, storage space, and good communications are also important. The method of transport should take into account urgency, mobilisation time, geographical factors, weather, traffic conditions, and cost.

Road transfer will be satisfactory for most patients. This also has the advantages of low cost, rapid mobilisation, less weather dependency, and easier patient monitoring. Air transfer should be considered for longer journeys (over about 50 miles (80 km) or 2 hours). The apparent speed must be balanced against organisational delays and transfer between vehicles at the beginning and end. Helicopters are recommended for journeys of 50-150 miles (80-240 km) or if access is difficult, but they provide a less comfortable environment than road ambulance or fixed wing aircraft, are expensive, and have a poorer safety record. Fixed wing aircraft, preferably pressurised, should be used for transfer distances over 150 miles (240 km).

Close liaison with local ambulance services is required. Contact numbers should be available in all intensive care units and accident and emergency departments to ensure rapid communication and advice.

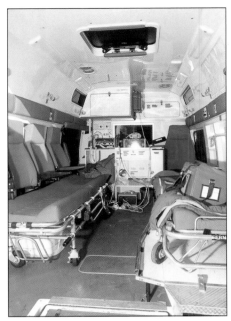

Comfort and safety of patients and staff are important

Equipment

Equipment must be robust, lightweight, and battery powered. The design of transport equipment has advanced greatly, and most hospitals now have the essentials. Many ambulance services also provide some items in standard ambulances.

Equipment for establishing and maintaining a safe airway is essential. Another prerequisite is a portable mechanical ventilator with disconnection alarms which can provide variable inspired oxygen concentrations, tidal volumes, respiratory rates, levels of positive end expiratory pressure, and inspiratory:expiratory ratios. The vehicle should carry sufficient oxygen to last the duration of the transfer plus a reserve of 1-2 hours.

A portable monitor with an illuminated display is required to record heart rhythm, oxygen saturation, blood pressure by non-invasive and invasive methods, end tidal carbon dioxide, and temperature. Alarms should be visible as well as audible because of extraneous noise during transfer. Suction equipment and a defibrillator should be available. A warming blanket is advantageous. The vehicle must also contain several syringe pumps with long battery life and appropriate drugs. A mobile phone for communication is advisable.

One person should be responsible for ensuring batteries are charged and supplies fully stocked. All those assisting in the transfer should know where the equipment is and be familiar with using the equipment and drugs.

If patients are transferred on standard ambulance trolleys equipment has to be carried by hand or laid on top of the patient, which is unsatisfactory. Special trolleys should be used that allow items to be secured to a pole or shelf above or below the patient.

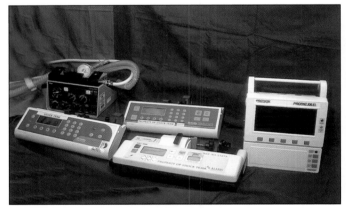

Portable ventilator, battery powered syringe pumps, and monitor

Accompanying staff

In addition to the vehicle's crew, a critically ill patient should be accompanied by a minimum of two attendants. One should be an experienced doctor competent in resuscitation, airway care, ventilation, and other organ support. The doctor, usually an anaesthetist, should ideally have training in intensive care, have

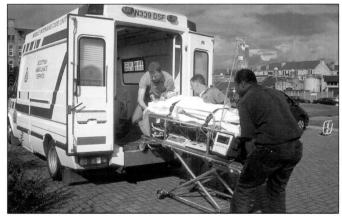

Trolley with shelf for equipment makes moving patients easier and safer

carried out previous transfers, and preferably have at least two years' postgraduate experience. He or she should be assisted by another doctor, nurse, paramedic, or technician familiar with intensive care procedures and equipment. Current staffing levels in many district general hospitals mean that this ideal is not always achievable.

The presence of experienced attendants will not only ensure that basics for ensuring safe transfer are undertaken but prevent transfers being rushed without full preparation; this often requires a senior voice. Hospitals should run regular training programmes in safe transport techniques.

Provision must be made for adequate insurance to cover death or disability of attendants in an accident during the course of their duties. The hospital trust should provide medical indemnity, and personal medical defence cover is also recommended.

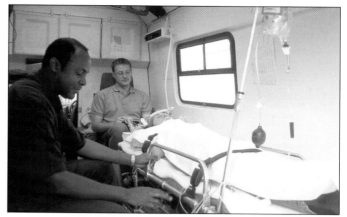

Patients should be accompanied by an experienced doctor and another trained member of staff

Preparation

Meticulous stabilisation of the patient before transfer is the key to avoiding complications during the journey. In addition to full clinical details and examination, monitoring before transfer should include electrocardiography, arterial oxygen saturation, (plus periodic blood gas analyses), blood pressure preferably by direct intra-arterial monitoring, central venous pressure where indicated, and urine output. Investigations should include chest radiography, other appropriate radiography or computed tomography, haematology, and biochemistry. If intra-abdominal bleeding is suspected the patient should have peritoneal lavage.

Intubating a patient in transit is difficult. If the patient is likely to develop a compromised airway or respiratory failure, he or she should be intubated before departure. Intubated patients should be mechanically ventilated. Inspired oxygen should be guided by arterial oxygen saturation and blood gas concentrations. Appropriate drugs should be used for sedation, analgesia, and muscle relaxation. A chest drain should be inserted if a pneumothorax is present or possible from fractured ribs.

Intravenous volume loading will usually be required to restore and maintain satisfactory blood pressure, perfusion, and urine output. Inotropic infusions may be needed. Unstable patients may need to have central venous pressure or pulmonary artery pressure monitored to optimise filling pressures and cardiac output. Hypovolaemic patients tolerate transfer poorly, and circulating volume should be normal or supranormal before transfer. A patient persistently hypotensive despite resuscitation must not be moved until all possible sources of continued blood loss have been identified and controlled. Unstable long bone fractures should be splinted to provide neurovascular protection.

It is important that these measures are not omitted in an attempt to speed transfer as resultant complications may be impossible to deal with once the journey has started.

A gastric drainage tube should be passed and all lines and tubes securely fixed. Equipment should be checked including battery charge and oxygen supply. Case notes, x ray films, a referral letter, and investigation reports should be prepared and blood or blood products collected. The receiving unit should be informed of the estimated time of arrival.

Travel arrangements should be discussed with relatives. They should not normally travel with the patient.

Transfer

Care should be maintained at the same level as in the intensive care unit, accepting that in transit it is almost impossible to

---

Is your patient ready for transfer?

Respiration
- Airway safe?
- Intubation and ventilation required?
- Sedation, analgesia, and paralysis adequate?
- Arterial oxygen pressure > 13 kPa? saturation > 95%?
- Arterial carbon dioxide pressure 4-5 kPa? (fit young adult)

Circulation
- Systolic blood pressure > 120 mm Hg?
- Heart rate < 120 beats/min?
- Perfusion OK?
- Intravenous access adequate?
- Circulating volume replaced?
- Blood needed?
- Urine volumes?
- Continuing bleeding? Site?

Head
- Glasgow coma score? Trend?
- Focal signs?
- Pupillary response?
- Skull fracture?

Other injuries
- Cervical spine, chest, ribs?
- Pneumothorax?
- Bleeding—intrathoracic or abdominal?
- Long bone or pelvic fractures?
- Adequate investigation?
- Adequate treatment?

Monitoring
- Electrocardiography?
- Pulse oximetry?
- Blood pressure?
- End tidal carbon dioxide pressure?
- Temperature?
- Central venous pressure, pulmonary artery pressure, or intracranial pressure needed?

Investigations
- Blood gases, biochemistry, and haematology sent?
- Correct radiographs taken?
- What else is needed? computed tomography, peritoneal lavage, laparotomy?

Departure checklist

- Do attendants have adequate experience, knowledge of case, clothing, insurance?
- Appropriate equipment and drugs?
- Batteries checked?
- Sufficient oxygen?
- Trolley available?
- Ambulance service aware or ready?
- Bed confirmed? Exact location?
- Case notes, x ray films, results, blood collected?
- Transfer chart prepared?
- Portable phone charged?
- Contact numbers known?
- Money or cards for emergencies?
- Estimated time of arrival notified?
- Return arrangements checked?
- Relatives informed?
- Patient stable, fully investigated?
- Monitoring attached and working?
- Drugs, pumps, lines rationalised and secured?
- Adequate sedation?
- Still stable after transfer to mobile equipment?
- Anything missed?

intervene. Monitoring of arterial oxygen saturation, expired carbon dioxide tensions, heart rhythm, temperature, and arterial pressure should be continuous. As non-invasive measurement of blood pressure is affected by movement, intra-arterial monitoring is recommended.

Transfer should be undertaken smoothly and not at high speed. A record must be maintained during transfer. Despite careful preparation unforeseen clinical emergencies may occur; the vehicle should then be stopped at the first safe opportunity to facilitate patient management.

Handover

On arrival there must be direct communication between the transfer team and the team who will assume responsibility for the patient. A record of the patient's history, treatment, and important events during transfer should be added to the notes. Radiographs, scans, and results of other investigations should be described and handed over. The transfer team should retain a record of the transfer on a prepared form for future audit.

The receiving hospital should provide refreshments and arrange for staff to return to base. Money or credit cards should be available for use in emergencies.

Audit, training, and funding

Regular audit of transfers is necessary to maintain and improve standards. The responsible consultant should review all transfers in and out of the hospital, and a similar process should be established at regional and national level.

Before taking responsibility for a transfer, staff should receive training and accompany patients as an observer. Resources are required to achieve this and to ensure safe transfer systems throughout the United Kingdom. Purchasers should reflect this in their budgetary priorities.

The patient transfer form was provided by ICBIS.

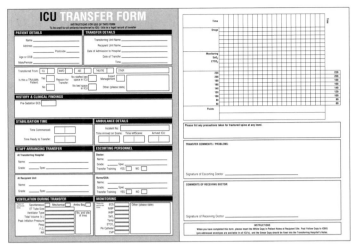

Form for recording patient transfer information

12   Recovery from intensive care

Richard D Griffiths, Christina Jones

Studies of outcome after intensive care suggest that death rates do not return to normal until 2-4 years after admission. Although some questionnaire studies have reported on morbidity, little published work exists on detailed clinical recovery or longer term residual effects of critical illness. The recovery process may present serious physical, psychological, and social problems for both patients and their families, and these may last for months or years. Although patients who have been in intensive care have often been extremely ill, been at high risk of death, and received care costing tens of thousands of pounds, detailed follow up and targeted support are still rare.

Discharge to the ward

Patients on mechanical ventilation are usually discharged from the intensive care unit to the ward when they can breathe unaided. However, several physical problems may still remain. Although these may not be serious enough to keep the patient in intensive care, if left untreated they could lead to readmission. Intensive care staff should therefore follow patients' progress on the ward for a few days to monitor recovery of multisystem disease and assure good continuity of care.

The commonest physical problem reported by intensive care patients is severe weakness and fatigue. Patients in intensive care can lose about 2% of muscle mass a day during their illness owing to a combination of primary muscle catabolism and atrophy secondary to neuropathic degeneration. They may lose over half their muscle mass, resulting in severe physical disability. Rebuilding such muscle losses can take over a year. Initially, patients may be so weak that they struggle to feed themselves, their cough power is greatly reduced, and they may have poor control of their swallowing and upper airways with a risk of aspiration. The nursing burden can be large. If patients can stand they are in danger of falling. This is often compounded by postural hypotension, which may reflect autonomic disturbances.

On discharge from intensive care patients may seem completely oriented and to understand the information they are given about their illness. Yet when questioned a few days later, many have little or no memory of their stay in intensive care or can remember only pain, suctioning, or lack of sleep. The only memories of some patients are nightmares, often of a persecutory nature in which they are subjected to torture, or paranoid delusions. These nightmares and delusions may be attributed to the illness, the use of opiate and sedative drugs, the unnatural environment of intensive care with its lack of a proper day and night, and to constant noise. Patients nursed in an intensive care unit without windows have even more unpleasant memories than those nursed in a unit with large windows.

The difficulty some patients have in accepting that the events in their dreams were not real is often not appreciated. In addition, patients are reluctant to tell ward staff about their nightmares for fear of being considered mad. However, confrontation, through discussion, of such problems allows patients to build up a coherent story rather than chaotic, intrusive memories and so put the experience behind them. The incidence of post-traumatic stress disorder is high after intensive care, and it is more common in patients who recall frightening adverse experiences.

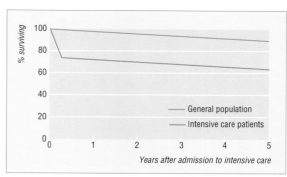

The 5 year mortality rate in intensive care patients is over 3 times that of the general population. However at 2 year survival rates are parallel. Adapted from Niskanen M et al. *Crit Care Med* 1996;24:1962-7.

Examples of physical disorders after intensive care

- Recovering organ failure (lung, kidney, liver etc)
- Severe muscle wasting and weakness including reduced cough power, pharyngeal weakness
- Joint stiffness
- Numbness, paraesthesia (peripheral neuropathy)
- Taste changes resulting in favourite foods being unpalatable
- Disturbances to sleep rhythm
- Cardiac and circulatory decompensation:
  Postural hypotension
- Reduced pulmonary reserve:
  Breathlessness on mild exertion
- Iatrogenic:
  Tracheal stenosis (for example, from repeated intubations)
  Nerve palsies (needle injuries)
  Scarring (needle and drain sites)

Taste changes and difficulties in feeding themselves may further compromise patients' nutritional state

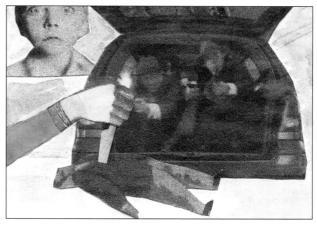

Intensive care patients often experience persecutory nightmares

43

When patients first see themselves in the mirror they may not recognise their face because of severe weight loss. With no memory of their illness, patients have no explanation for this frightening confrontation, and they may also find it difficult to appreciate why they feel so awful. For example, they may only remember coming in for elective surgery and waking up on the ward, seemingly the next morning, and be left thinking "why have I lost all this weight, why am I so weak?"

Discharge home

It is often when patients go home that they realise how debilitated they are; commonly, they cannot climb stairs. Relatives take on the care of the patients and, for example, report sleeplessness because of worry about whether the patient is still breathing. Relatives often report that patients are hard to live with because of irritability and impatience with the slowness of their recovery.

Many healthcare professionals believe that it is better for patients not to remember their intensive care stay. This means that patients are unable to explain why they feel so debilitated. Although the family may try to explain, the lack of a concrete memory makes it difficult for patients to realise just how ill they have been and just how long it will take them to recover. Patients consequently have unrealistic expectations of recovery and think in terms of weeks instead of months, if not years.

Except for very elderly and some trauma and neurological patients, most intensive care patients will not receive any physiotherapy once they are able to walk unaided in hospital. However, muscle loss and peripheral neuropathies may affect their balance, and they have poor ability to right themselves. Walking unaided outside in icy conditions or in a wind is potentially dangerous and frightening for the patient. In addition, minor physical problems such as hair loss, skin dryness, or fingernail ridges, which often occur after critical illness can be particularly distressing because of the lack of an adequate explanation during the discharge process.

Two months to one year

Physical problems related to muscle weakness are still common 2 months after intensive care and can still be seen at 6 months. These problems often affect self care activities such as climbing stairs, getting out of the bath, turning off taps, driving a car, and returning to work. Fear of falling and being unable to get up again is common.

The prolonged recovery period leads to several problems, and intensive care survivors experience considerable levels of depression and anxiety. Patients often avoid company and show less affection to their partners. In one study 45% of patients questioned at 6 months reported going out less often, 41% took part in fewer social activities, and a quarter reported being irritable with their relatives.

Coupled to this social isolation is a dependence on others to make decisions and a tendency towards being obstinate. Patients also report feeling overwhelmed in crowded places or being afraid to go out alone. Some patients describe full blown panic attacks, although they may not necessarily recognise them as such. The longer panic attacks are left untreated, the more refractory they are likely to be. Long term treatment is needed by 36-40% of people with panic attacks presenting for help.

Patients understandably feel that the recovery phase of their critical illness is the most stressful period as they have to come to terms with how ill and close to death they have been. The presence of social support increases tolerance to stressful

Patient's view

A 42 year old woman with acute pancreatitis required a 40 day stay in intensive care. She had been ill in hospital for several weeks before transfer. When she went home she found she had lost 2 months from her memory—the time in intensive care and in the ward before that. She worried about what had happened to her and why she could not remember.

She learnt about her illness and why she could not remember at the follow up clinic. She was relieved that there was nothing wrong with her mind and that it is common not to be able to remember.

Relative's view

After John's wife had been in intensive care he felt that it was better that she didn't know about her illness and so wouldn't discuss it. He had been very upset and wanted to protect her. He could not bring himself to return to hospital, even to accompany his wife to outpatient clinics. His wife was initially upset by this behaviour. However, once she had been told how ill she had been she understood how much stress John had been under and his subsequent behaviour.

Psychological disorders
- Depression:
  Anger and conflict with the family
- Anxiety:
  Are they going to get back to normal?
  Panic attacks
  Fear of dying
- Guilt
- Recurrent nightmares
- Post traumatic stress disorder

Actual examples of problems reported by patients
"I get panicky if I go out alone in case I am taken ill"
"I get very angry with my family. They keep fussing when I try to do things for myself"
"I feel very angry with myself for not being back to normal by now"
"I've tried to help by doing the washing up but I keep dropping the crockery"
"When I first went home I climbed the stairs on my hands and knees and came down on my bottom"
"I don't want to go to sleep because I keep dreaming that I'm back in ICU"
"My whole time in ICU I dreamt I had been kidnapped and locked in the boot of a car"
"I feel very guilty when I think about what my family has been through"

situations and has, in general, a beneficial effect on health. Social isolation, however, seems to act as a source of chronic stress. Much of the impact caused by life events may be the result of the profound changes they produce in social relationships.

Rehabilitation after critical illness

Early intervention is needed to prevent physical and psychological problems. This should ideally start when the patient is moved to the ward. Activity is the key to recovery, but the overwhelming weakness that patients report as they start to recover and the length of the convalescent process means that they require considerable determination to exercise. Most patients have little idea how and when to start exercising or how to pace themselves.

Simply giving intensive care patients a discharge booklet outlining possible problems they might encounter during their recovery has proved unsuccessful. Despite using a booklet, 25% of patients attending an intensive care follow up clinic scored highly for anxiety and depression 2 months after intensive care.

Good support after intensive care is essential

Guide to care after hospital discharge

Integration of physical and psychological care is clearly in the best interest of these patients. What issues need to be addressed when planning for hospital discharge for intensive care patients? A partnership is needed between the patient's general practitioner, ward doctor, and intensive care doctor. Clear information about the illness should be provided to patients, their families, and their general practitioners. Patients need to be given some idea about how long it will take them to recover. Both patients and their families should be given the opportunity to be debriefed about the illness, the time in intensive care, and what it means, preferably by staff who were involved in the patients' care. Debriefing should tackle not only the reasons for admission to intensive care and events while they were there but also any distorted memories patients may have. For many patients, simply knowing that nightmares and paranoid delusions are normal after critical illness is sufficient for them to put the memories in context.

It is helpful to outline a plan with patients and their families for convalescence and rehabilitation. Patients should have access to referral to specialists such as clinical psychologists and dieticians. Work, particularly in cardiac rehabilitation, suggests that providing written information about critical illness, self help advice to manage the typical problems patients might face during recovery, and an exercise programme may be helpful.

Guide for care after discharge

- Initial review by intensive care staff to ensure medical and nursing handover is thorough, seamless, and continuous
- Early explanation of illness to patient, preferably with a relative present to ensure uniformity of experience
- Advice to patients on problems and information on the time scale of recovery
- Reinforcement of the patients' responsibility for their recovery
- Practical advice on rehabilitation, exercise, and nutrition
- Detailed letter to general practitioner detailing patients' illness
- Early recognition and diagnosis of physical and psychological problems in patients and relatives
- Follow up for at least 6 months after discharge from hospital that reviews not only the patient's physical problems but also psychological issues for patients and close relatives

---

13 Cutting edge

Mervyn Singer, Rod Little

Few areas of clinical medicine are changing as rapidly as intensive care. Greater understanding of the pathophysiology of disease processes, technological innovations, targeted pharmaceutical and "nutriceutical" interventions, and the use of specialised audit and scoring methods to improve patient classification and monitor disease progression have all contributed to changes in practice in the past decade. This article considers developments that may affect patient management in the next 10 years.

Prevention

There is an increasing appreciation of the need to prevent critical illness with proactive care rather than to offer reactive support once organ failure is established. This has considerable resource implications, although savings should be made through reduced requirement for intensive care. Emphasis should be placed on identifying patients at risk, with early recognition of physiological disturbances and prompt correction to avoid subsequent major complications.

Maintenance of organ perfusion
The concept of a perioperative tissue oxygen debt resulting in organ dysfunction, which need not be clinically manifest until several days after an operation, is now accepted. Many high risk patients cannot mount an adequate haemodynamic response to the stress of surgery, and this may be compounded by unrecognised hypovolaemia and poor organ perfusion. Tissue hypoxia and reperfusion injury both fuel the subsequent systemic inflammatory response.

Several recent studies have shown a strong relation between intraoperative haemodynamic deterioration and postoperative complications. Significant improvements in outcome and reductions in hospital stay have been achieved by optimising perioperative circulatory function using fluid loading with or without vasoactive drugs, and guided by monitoring of cardiac output.

Ward supervision
The hospital mortality of patients admitted to intensive care from general wards (40-45%) is significantly higher than that of patients admitted directly from either accident and emergency (30%) or the operating theatre (20%). This is partly because of delays in recognising problems and suboptimal treatment.

Attempts are being made to improve patient care in general wards and thereby pre-empt the need for intensive care. The Liverpool Hospital in New South Wales, Australia, has recently pioneered medical emergency teams. These are expert teams that can be called by medical or nursing staff when patients meet predetermined physiological criteria or give cause for concern. The high dependency unit is also being proposed as a means of improving the management of high risk patients.

Immunological and genetic manipulation
Individual susceptibility to the effects of inflammatory activation may be determined genetically, and this raises the possibility of assessment before procedures such as major elective surgery. For example, septic patients homozygous for the tumour necrosis factor B2 allele had higher plasma tumour necrosis

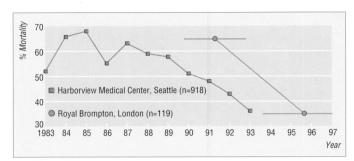

Outcome from acute respiratory distress syndrome has improved over the past 15 years. Data from Milberg JA et al. Improved survival of patients with acute respiratory distress syndrome. *JAMA* 1995;306-9 and Abel SJ et al. Reduced mortality in association with the acute respiratory distress syndrome. *Thorax* 1998;53:292-4

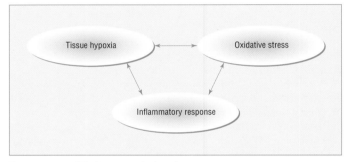

Factors responsible for organ dysfunction

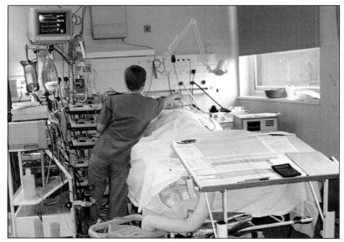

Outcome from intensive care is related to source of admission

46

factor-α concentrations, organ failure scores, and mortality than heterozygous septic patients. Drugs may be developed to boost or suppress the inflammatory response in high risk patients.

The degree of acquired endogenous immunity may also be important. For example, patients with high titres of endogenous endotoxin antibodies have better outcomes after cardiac surgery; passive or active immunisation programmes may therefore be effective.

Pharmaceutical advances

Modulating the inflammatory response

Patients may develop (multiple) organ dysfunction after insults such as infection and trauma. Increasing awareness of the roles of endotoxin and other toxins; endogenous proinflammatory, vasoactive, and anti-inflammatory mediators; tissue hypoxia; and subsequent reperfusion injury has led to drugs targeted against these pathophysiological mechanisms.

Most effort to date has been expended on modulating the inflammatory response with immunotherapeutic drugs aimed against endotoxins or mediators such as the cytokines, tumour necrosis factor, and interleukin-1. Unfortunately, the promising results shown in both laboratory and small patient groups have yet to be reproduced in large multicentre trials. Paradoxically, this has helped to clarify some of the problems of study design that exist when looking at such a heterogeneous population. But many other issues remain—for instance, when to give the drug and the balance between blocking and enhancing the inflammatory response. These difficulties are compounded by enormous variation in the pattern of response between patients. This variation may be due to coexisting illness or to genetic predisposition.

In future there may be targeted treatment guided by appropriate immunological markers which can be measured at the bedside. Identification of genetically high risk patients will allow them to have closer monitoring, and drugs may also be developed to modulate their inflammatory response.

Reducing cellular injury

Recognition of the importance of hypoxia in the pathogenesis of cellular injury has stimulated development of various drugs that are either protective or augment tissue oxygenation—for example, by shifting the oxyhaemoglobin dissociation curve or enhancing cellular oxygen use. Specific channels, receptors, and signalling pathways are activated by tissue hypoxia; antagonism or stimulation of these may prove beneficial.

Treatments are also being developed to prevent the damage caused to cell membranes, protein, DNA, and mitochondria by raised intracellular concentrations of calcium and excessive production of reactive oxygen and nitrogen species (superoxide, hydroxyl radical, nitric oxide, etc).

Modifying vascular tone and function

Nitric oxide is associated with profound hypotension in hyperinflammatory syndromes such as sepsis. Inhibitors of the synthesising enzyme (nitric oxide synthase) or its effector pathways have been well studied. A recent large multicentre study of a nitric oxide synthase inhibitor was, however, terminated prematurely because of adverse outcome. Nevertheless, drugs that modify vascular tone and the microcirculation by acting on the endothelium (including leucocyte and platelet interactions), smooth muscle tone, and rheology could optimise microvascular distribution of blood flow and tissue perfusion, thereby reducing tissue damage.

In the long term, a cocktail of the agents described above, rather than any single drug, is likely to be used to prevent,

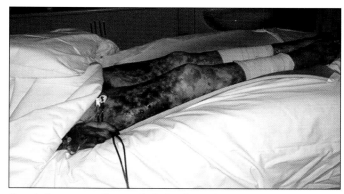

Genetic factors may affect survival of patients with septicaemia

---

Some immunotherapeutic drugs tested in randomised, controlled phase II or III trials in human sepsis

- Methylprednisolone
- Hyperimmune immunoglobulin
- Endotoxin antibody
- Bactericidal permeability increasing protein
- Tumour necrosis factor antibody
- Soluble tumour necrosis factor receptor antibody
- Interleukin-1 receptor antagonist
- Platelet activating factor antagonists
- Bradykinin antagonists
- Ibuprofen
- Antithrombin III
- Activated protein c
- N-acetyl cysteine
- Procysteine
- Nitric oxide synthase inhibitor (L-monomethyl N^G-arginine (L-NMMA))

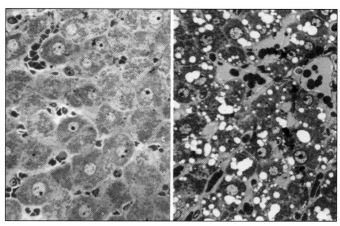

Effects of hypoxia on rat liver

Other drugs being tried in intensive care

- Drugs to improve gas exchange
- Sedatives or analgesics that are short acting despite prolonged administration
- Specific vasoactive drugs
- Neuroprotective drugs for use after neurosurgery or cardiothoracic surgery, head trauma, or cardiorespiratory arrest
- New antibiotics to deal with increasingly multiresistant micro-organisms
- Anabolic hormones (some with immunomodulatory effects) such as growth factors which can hasten rehabilitation

attenuate, or treat hypoxic, infectious, and other insults that lead to multiple organ failure.

Blood substitutes

Artificial haemoglobin and fluorocarbon solutions carry much higher amounts of oxygen than equivalent volumes of standard plasma or crystalloid solutions. These have been in development for several decades as an alternative to blood in emergency situations and peroperatively (for example, for Jehovah's witnesses). Problems such as nephrotoxicity and inadequate release of oxygen to tissues have delayed their introduction into routine use, although recent advances have largely overcome these difficulties—for example, diasprin cross linkage of haemoglobin molecules and liposome encapsulation. Multicentre trials are now in progress in various potential applications. The first artifical haemoglobins are likely to be commercially available within a year.

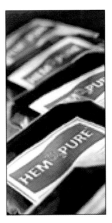

Blood substitutes will be available shortly for clinical care

Ventilation and gas exchange

The increasing use of mechanical ventilation was the driving force behind the creation of intensive care units. Over the past 30 years ventilators have become more sophisticated, with various techniques incorporated to minimise iatrogenic trauma and facilitate patients' tolerance and weaning. Particular attention has been applied to non-invasive modes of ventilation such as biphasic positive airways ventilation through a nasal or face mask, high frequency oscillation, and negative pressure ventilation with a cuirass ventilator. Continued developments will reduce the need for tracheal intubation—for example, in those with acute-on-chronic respiratory failure. Computer controlled ventilation, in which the ventilator constantly adjusts to changes in lung compliance and blood gas measurements, is another recent development.

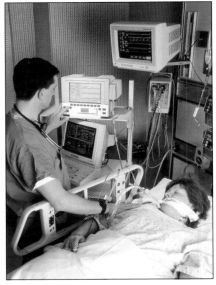

Continuous intra-arterial blood gas monitoring

There has also been considerable enthusiasm for locally applied agents that improve gas exchange or reduce lung injury. These include inhaled nitric oxide, nebulised epoprostenol, and nebulised artificial surfactants. Although these agents produce short term improvement in many patients with acute respiratory failure, only surfactants in neonatal respiratory distress have been shown to improve outcome. A novel concept is to attenuate the degree of lung fibrosis in conditions such as the acute respiratory distress syndrome by using specific inhibitors instilled into the lung—for example, thrombin inhibitors.

Finally, trials of liquid ventilation are ongoing. The lungs are filled with a fluorocarbon to functional residual capacity—that is, when a fluid meniscus is seen in the endotracheal tube on end expiration—and are ventilated through this medium. Early results have been highly encouraging in terms of gas exchange, bronchial lavage, surfactant-like properties, and anti-inflammatory properties and suggest that the technique will improve outcome.

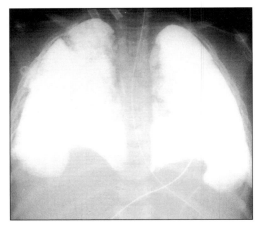

Radiograph of patient receiving liquid ventilation

Nutrition

Increasing awareness of the importance of nutrition and avoiding malnutrition has encouraged earlier introduction of feeding for critically ill patients. Recent laboratory studies have shown various nutrients to have positive immunomodulatory effects, including glutamine, polyunsaturated fatty acids, and arginine. "Immunoenhanced" diets have been given to intensive care patients, surgical patients, burn patients, and those having bone marrow transplantation. Reduced morbidity and,

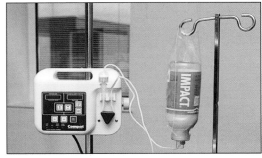

Immunonutrition

occasionally, mortality have been shown, although confirmatory large scale multicentre studies are awaited.

Other areas under investigation include the concept of protecting the gastrointestinal surface with probiotic bacteria. Shortening the catabolic phase of injury and enhancing anabolism by infusion of growth hormone and insulin growth factor-1 was recently tested but produced an adverse outcome.

Monitoring

Treatment in intensive care should always be guided by adequate monitoring. Advances have enabled cardiorespiratory function to be monitored continuously and, increasingly, by non-invasive or minimally invasive techniques. These techniques are being continually refined and some are now being commercially marketed. Further efforts are being made to measure regional organ perfusion (and its adequacy) through tissue or arteriovenous oxygen or carbon dioxide pressure, lactate concentration, or other markers such as the cytochrome aa_3 redox state, and hepatic clearance of indocyanine green.

Although the importance of raised plasma concentrations of circulating inflammatory mediators such as interleukin-6 and procalcitonin is not yet fully understood, kits are being developed to allow measurement at the bedside. The results may be used to predict sepsis or to indicate the correct timing for giving immunomodulating drugs.

Finally, paperless monitoring with sophisticated computers interfaced with physiological monitors, fluid infusion pumps and drainage sets, pathology laboratories, and pharmacy should not only facilitate data collection and patient management but provide a sophisticated and comprehensive database for audit and research. Early versions are already in operation in over 100 intensive care units worldwide, but continual refinement and technological advances should produce widespread uptake of these systems.

Audit, guidelines, and evidence based medicine

The scoring systems for physiological abnormality, therapeutic intervention, organ dysfunction, and predicting outcome are far more complex than in any other specialty. Indeed, many intensive care units are now employing dedicated audit staff to collect these data. The data are being incorporated into national and international databases, enabling better definition of patient populations and disease progression. Variations in case mix between units are being taken into account, and this will allow quality issues to be explored in far greater detail than at present.

Clinical governance is likely to lead to local, regional, national, or even international, practice guidelines. These will be evidence based where possible. However, the current paucity of conclusive large scale, randomised controlled trial data, and the logistical, ethical, and financial difficulties in conducting such studies, will often oblige these to be consensus led.

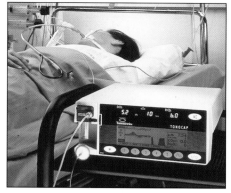

Measurement of gastric mucosal pco_2, a marker of organ perfusion

Examples of new monitoring techniques

Variable	Monitoring
Arterial blood gas concentrations and pH	Continuous by intra-arterial catheters Intermittent by portable devices
Cardiac output	Intraoesophageal probes, surface electrodes, or via radial arterial cannulas
Gastric mucosal carbon dioxide pressure (index of tissue perfusion)	Continuous through nasogastric catheter

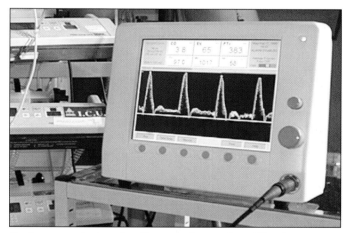

Continuous monitoring of cardiac output by oesophageal Doppler ultrasonograph

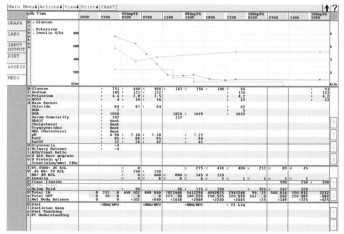

Computerised monitoring system

The radiograph was provided by Dr R Hirschl, the oesophageal Doppler monitor by Deltex, continuous air tonometer by Datex-Ohmeda, the picture of the computerised monitoring system by Hewlett Packard, and the blood gas analyser by Diametrics

Index

Page numbers in italics refer to illustrations.